Loving Someone with Frontotemporal Dementia

A Partner's Guide to Understanding Personality Changes, Maintaining Connection, and Caring for Yourself

Lawrence Louis Cowan

This book is intended for informational and educational purposes only. It does not constitute medical, legal, financial, or psychological advice. The information provided should not be used as a substitute for consultation with qualified healthcare providers, attorneys, financial planners, or mental health professionals. Always seek the guidance of a licensed professional regarding any medical condition, legal matter, or financial decision.

No guarantees or warranties are made regarding the accuracy, completeness, or applicability of any information contained in this book. Individual circumstances vary, and outcomes depend on many factors outside the scope of this publication. The author and publisher disclaim any liability for actions taken or not taken based on the content of this book.

Any names, characters, and scenarios used in this book are composites drawn from clinical knowledge, published research, and general caregiving experience. They are not intended to represent any specific individual, living or deceased. Any resemblance to actual persons is coincidental and unintentional. No example or scenario is intended to harm, misrepresent, or identify any person or entity.

First Edition:2026

ISBN: 978-1-7646697-8-8

Table of Contents

Preface

Frontotemporal dementia is the most common cause of dementia in people under sixty-five, yet it remains one of the least understood neurodegenerative diseases in public awareness and in primary care practice. The average time from first symptom to correct diagnosis exceeds three years. During those years, the person with FTD is frequently misdiagnosed with depression, bipolar disorder, or marital dysfunction, while the partner who first noticed the changes is frequently dismissed. The diagnoses of Bruce Willis and Wendy Williams brought the term into public conversation, and Emma Heming Willis's 2025 memoir demonstrated that demand for FTD caregiver content is enormous. What no English-language bookshelf currently holds is a structured, practical guide written specifically for the spouse or long-term partner.

Frontotemporal dementia is not Alzheimer's disease. It targets the frontal and anterior temporal lobes, the regions responsible for personality, social behavior, empathy, judgment, and language. Memory is often preserved well into the disease, which is precisely why it evades detection. The result is a clinical picture that looks, from the outside, less like illness and more like a person choosing to become cruel, reckless, or indifferent. For the partner, this distinction between personality change and memory loss is not academic. It shapes every interaction, every care decision, and every dimension of grief.

The gap this book addresses is specific. Existing FTD literature falls into three categories: personal memoirs that document one family's experience without offering transferable guidance, clinical textbooks written for neurologists and researchers, and brief self-published summaries that reviewers consistently describe as superficial. No title currently available provides the partner with a chapter-by-chapter framework covering behavioral management strategies grounded in the neuroscience of frontal lobe damage, communication techniques validated for primary progressive aphasia, the legal and financial architecture that must be built while cognitive capacity remains, and the particular form of grief, described by Pauline Boss as ambiguous loss, that accompanies loving someone who is physically present and psychologically receding.

This book supplies that framework. It is organized around the actual arc of the disease as experienced by the care partner: from the pre-diagnosis years through behavioral and language changes, financial and safety planning, family communication, the placement decision, hospice advocacy, and reconstruction after death. Each chapter follows a consistent structure that includes clinical content, perspective sidebars for both the person with FTD and the supporting partner, ready-to-use scripts for conversations with medical teams and family members, and low-demand reflection prompts. The approach is grounded in current FTD research, the work of specialists at centers including UCSF, the University of Pennsylvania, and the Association for Frontotemporal Degeneration, and the reported experience of hundreds of care partners across published studies and clinical practice.

The primary reader is the spouse or long-term partner of someone with any FTD subtype, including behavioral variant FTD, all three forms of primary progressive aphasia, and FTD with motor features. Adult children, siblings, therapists, social workers, and pastoral care providers will also find the content applicable, though the voice throughout speaks to the person sharing a life and a home with the diagnosis.

This book is not a substitute for a neurologist, an elder law attorney, a genetic counselor, or a licensed therapist. It does not promise to slow the disease or to eliminate the grief that accompanies it. It is a practical guide built to reduce the distance between diagnosis and competent action, so that the years ahead are shaped by information rather than improvisation.

PART ONE: UNDERSTANDING WHAT IS HAPPENING

The first part of this book is about the ground underneath you. Before you can figure out what to do, you need a reasonable map of what you are dealing with. These four chapters cover the terrain from the first strange moments through the diagnosis appointment and into the single most important reframe you will ever make about your person.

You do not need to read these chapters in order. If you are still in the pre-diagnosis fog, start with Chapter 1. If you walked out of a neurologist's office this week, start with Chapter 3. If you are months in and you keep finding yourself furious at someone you love, open to Chapter 4.

Whatever brought you here, you are not behind. You are not failing. You are learning something almost nobody around you knows.

Chapter 1. When Something Feels Wrong

Linda kept a Google Doc on her phone called "Things." She started it the night her husband Richard made a cruel joke at their daughter's engagement party about the groom's weight. Richard had never made jokes like that in thirty years of marriage. He was a gentle man. He cried at commercials. He apologized to the dog when he stepped on her tail.

That night, after the party, she sat in the closet with the door closed so Richard would not hear her, and she typed the date and a single sentence: "Richard said something mean to Kevin tonight and it was like watching a stranger use his mouth."

Over the next two years, the document grew. Richard stopped caring about the garden he had tended for a decade. He ate entire bags of licorice in a sitting. He laughed, once, at a news story about a child pulled dead from a swimming pool. He bought three identical cordless drills on the same Amazon order and could not explain why. He told a woman at the grocery store that her dress was too tight. He forgot the word for "spatula," then "fork," then remembered them ten minutes later as if nothing had happened.

Linda took the document to Richard's primary care doctor. The doctor read three entries and said, warmly, that men go through things in their sixties. He asked Richard if he was drinking more. He asked Linda if the marriage was okay. He suggested couples counseling and a low-dose antidepressant for Richard.

Linda went home and added a new entry: "Dr. P. thinks I am the problem."

It would be another eighteen months before a neurologist, reading the same document, would say the words "frontotemporal dementia" out loud. By then the document had 114 entries. Linda had typed each one in the closet.

You may already have a document like Linda's. It might live in your Notes app, or in a notebook in your nightstand drawer, or only in your head. You might have shown parts of it to friends, to family, to a doctor, and been told you are exaggerating, or stressed, or menopausal, or that you just need a vacation. You may have started to wonder if the problem is actually you.

The problem is not you. Your gut noticed before any scan could.

Chapter Principle

In frontotemporal dementia, the partner is almost always the first person to know something is wrong, and almost always the last person to be believed. The years between those two facts are some of the loneliest of your life. This chapter is about what to do with what you already see.

1.1 The Subtle Shift You Alone Can See

FTD does not announce itself. It does not show up the way Alzheimer's does in the movies, with someone forgetting their grandchildren's names or getting lost on their own street. FTD starts with personality changes, and personality changes are the hardest thing in the world to prove.

Your person becomes a little more short-tempered. A little less patient with the grandkids. A little more willing to spend money you do not have on something you do not need. A little less interested in the hobby they loved. A little quieter at dinner. A little cruder at parties. A little colder when your mother died.

Each change, in isolation, is something you can explain away. People change. Marriages go through phases. Sixty-year-olds get cranky. A midlife crisis is a real thing. A stressful job takes a toll.

What you see, that nobody else can see, is the pattern. You have lived with this person for years or decades. You know the exact rhythm of their laugh. You know what they look like when they are worried, when they are lying, when they are trying to be polite. You are the only human being on earth with a baseline for comparison. When that baseline starts to shift, you feel it in your body before you understand it in your head.

Research on FTD confirms what you already suspect. The average time from first symptom to correct diagnosis is generally reported to exceed three years. During those years, the person with FTD typically sees multiple providers, receives multiple incorrect diagnoses, and is often treated for depression, bipolar disorder, anxiety, or other psychiatric conditions before anyone considers a neurodegenerative cause (Onyike & Diehl-Schmid, 2013). The partner, meanwhile, is often asked if they might be the one with the problem.

This is not a failure of medicine in some abstract sense. It is a structural feature of how FTD presents. The early changes look exactly like life. Doctors do not run brain scans for rudeness.

1.2 Why Doctors Often Miss It First

There are concrete reasons physicians miss FTD in the early stages, and understanding those reasons will help you advocate.

First, most primary care doctors see perhaps one or two cases of FTD in their entire career. It is a rare disease. The disease they see every week is depression, and early bvFTD (behavioral variant FTD) can look almost identical to depression: reduced interest, flat mood, social withdrawal, reduced motivation. The standard screening tools catch depression. They do not catch FTD.

Second, standard cognitive screens like the Mini-Mental State Examination or the Montreal Cognitive Assessment are designed to catch Alzheimer's. They test memory and orientation. Someone with early bvFTD can ace them. Your husband can score a 29 out of 30 on a MoCA and still come home and shoplift at a gas station the same afternoon.

Third, the person with FTD is often unaware of their own changes. This is not denial. It is a core symptom of the disease called anosognosia, a neurological loss of insight produced by the same frontal lobe damage causing the behavior. When the doctor asks your husband if anything is wrong, he will say no. And he will mean it. He is not lying to you. He genuinely cannot see what you see.

Fourth, FTD is most common in people aged 45 to 65, which means the presumed explanation is almost always something age-appropriate: stress, midlife crisis, depression, a marriage problem, a new job, aging itself. The neurological explanation is ranked low on the differential.

Fifth, and this one is worth naming plainly, some doctors default to distrusting the wife when the husband is still articulate, and sometimes the husband when the wife is still articulate. Your partner shows up for the fifteen-minute appointment, performs well, cracks a joke, and the doctor mirrors that confidence back at you. This is not conscious sexism or dismissal in most cases. It is a cognitive shortcut that happens to fail catastrophically in FTD.

1.3 What Separates FTD From Midlife Crisis

You will probably be told that what you are seeing is a midlife crisis. It is worth knowing how to tell the difference.

A midlife crisis is usually about the person trying to feel something. They buy the motorcycle because they want to feel young. They have the affair because they want to feel wanted. They quit the corporate job because they want to feel alive. The behaviors are unwise, often harmful, and frequently regrettable, but they trace back to a felt need and the person can articulate that need.

FTD behaviors do not trace back to anything. Your husband does not buy three identical drills because he wants to feel like a craftsman. He buys them because the impulse arose and nothing in his brain stopped it. Ask him why and he will say, honestly, "I don't know." He cannot construct a retrospective reason because there was no reason. The filter that would have stopped the purchase is not working. That is it.

A midlife crisis usually shows up with increased emotional intensity. FTD usually shows up with reduced emotional intensity. The midlife-crisis husband cries about feeling trapped. The FTD husband does not cry about anything, including his mother's funeral. A midlife crisis involves a rearrangement of priorities. FTD involves a flattening of priorities. The person stops caring about the hobby they loved, but they also stop caring about the new thing that was supposed to replace it.

A midlife crisis responds to conversation. FTD does not. If you sit your partner down, lay out your concerns, and they promise to do better, and then three weeks later nothing has changed and they have forgotten the conversation ever happened, you are not looking at a midlife crisis.

1.4 Keeping a Behavior Log That Doctors Will Respect

Linda's Google Doc was, in retrospect, the most important thing she did in those two years. It was also the thing that eventually got Richard seen.

A good behavior log has four qualities. It is contemporaneous, meaning you write things down within a day or two of noticing them, not from memory six months later. It is specific, meaning it records exact quotes, exact purchases, exact amounts, exact dates, not general impressions. It is observational, meaning it describes what you saw rather than what you interpreted. And it is cumulative, meaning it accrues over months in a way that shows a pattern rather than a single bad day.

A single entry might read: "March 12. Richard told the server at dinner her accent was 'hard to listen to.' She looked upset. He did not apologize or notice. Ten years ago he would have been mortified."

That kind of entry, across a document of a hundred like it, is almost impossible for a doctor to dismiss. It is the difference between "I think my husband is acting strange" and "Here are forty-three instances of specific uncharacteristic behavior over the past fourteen months, in chronological order, with dates."

Action Challenge

If you do not already have a behavior log, start one today. Open a Note on your phone, title it something neutral like "Household Log" or "Notes," and add three entries from the past week. Do not wait until you have time. You do not have time. Five minutes is enough.

1.5 Getting a Referral to a Cognitive Neurologist

The person you need is not a general neurologist. It is not a psychiatrist. It is not a geriatrician, though one may help you get the referral. The person you need is a behavioral or cognitive neurologist, ideally at an academic medical center with a memory and aging program.

Ask your primary care provider for a referral specifically to a behavioral neurology clinic or a memory disorders clinic. If they hesitate, say this, verbatim: "I am concerned about early-onset neurodegenerative disease. I would like a referral to a memory clinic for evaluation." The word "neurodegenerative" shifts the conversation. Some providers will still push back. If yours does, find another provider.

Bring the behavior log to the first appointment. Bring photographs or, better, short video clips of changed behavior if you have any. Bring a list of medications your partner is taking. Bring someone else with you if you can, because you will not remember everything you hear. If there is a teenage or adult child who has noticed changes, ask if they can write a short letter describing what they have observed. Outside corroboration lands differently than a spouse alone.

Expect the evaluation to take hours, or across multiple visits. Expect blood work, brain imaging (usually MRI, sometimes PET), neuropsychological testing. Expect the neurologist to ask your partner questions in front of you and to ask you questions while your partner is in the room. Expect, at some point, to be asked to step out so they can interview your partner alone. Expect all of this to be exhausting.

Expect, also, not to get a definitive diagnosis on day one. FTD is a clinical diagnosis, sometimes supported by imaging and occasionally by genetic testing, and the process takes time. A good neurologist will tell you what they are ruling in and ruling out, not hand you a name on the first visit.

What you are looking for from the first appointment is this: the word "frontotemporal" spoken out loud, even as a possibility to investigate. That word is the door. Once it has been said by a specialist, everything else becomes easier to access.

From the Person with FTD's Perspective

Before diagnosis, when insight is still partially present, many people with FTD describe a vague sense that something is not right, without being able to name what. Some write in journals about feeling "less like myself." Some tell their spouse, once, something like "I don't know why I did that." These moments pass quickly and are rarely repeated, because the capacity to reflect on one's own behavior is one of the earliest things the disease takes.

By the time the neurologist sees them, most people with FTD do not feel anything is wrong. This is not denial. It is the disease. The frontal lobe, which is the part of the brain that lets you watch yourself and judge your own behavior, is precisely the part that is shrinking. Your person is not refusing to see what you see. They are, at a biological level, unable to.

Holding this is one of the hardest things about loving someone with FTD. You will want them to agree with you. You will want them to confirm your reality. They cannot. The absence of their confirmation is not evidence that your reality is wrong. It is evidence of the disease.

From the Supporting Partner's Perspective

You have been the only one who sees this for a long time. You have probably doubted yourself more in the last year than in the rest of your life combined. You have wondered if you are overreacting, if you are making things up, if you are the problem. You have cried in parking lots. You have lain awake running through instances. You have second-guessed yourself every time your partner has a good day.

None of that is weakness. All of it is rational. You are being asked to trust a perception no one around you confirms, while the evidence accumulates in a shape only you can see. Your nervous system has been doing the work that a medical system should have been doing, and it has been doing it alone.

It will help you, over time, to say out loud the sentence you may not have let yourself say yet: "Something is wrong with my partner, and it is not about our marriage." That sentence will become a kind of spine. You may need to say it to yourself before anyone else believes it.

Practical Strategies and Scripts

If your partner's primary care doctor dismisses your concerns: "I hear you that a lot of this can look like depression or stress. I would like to rule out a neurological cause before we try an antidepressant. Can you refer us to a memory clinic or behavioral neurologist for evaluation?"

If your partner refuses to go to the appointment: "The kids would feel better if we both got checkups this year. I made us both appointments. I'll go first." Then schedule your partner's appointment on the same day at the same clinic. Framing it as a shared event rather than a focused assessment of them is often the only way into the door.

If a family member accuses you of exaggerating: "I don't need you to believe me about the diagnosis. I need you to stop telling me I'm imagining it. We'll know more after the next appointment." Do not argue. Restate and exit.

If you need to describe what you are seeing to a doctor in under two minutes: "Over the past [time frame], I have observed specific, uncharacteristic changes in my spouse's behavior, including [three concrete examples]. These are out of character and have been getting more frequent. I am concerned about an underlying medical cause."

Reflection Prompts

Take these only if you want them. Skip any that do not fit. There are no wrong answers.

What was the first moment you thought, "something is wrong"? Where were you? What did you notice?

Who in your life knows some version of what you are seeing? Who have you not told, and why?

What would you need to be able to believe your own perception without waiting for a doctor to confirm it?

If a trusted friend described your last year to you, what would you tell them to do?

The Quick Version

FTD starts with personality changes, not memory loss, which is why it is almost always missed in the early years. The partner sees it first, because the partner is the only person with a baseline to compare against. Doctors often misdiagnose FTD as depression, midlife crisis, or marital problems for years before it is named correctly. A specific, dated, contemporaneous behavior log is the single most effective tool for getting taken seriously. The specialist you want is a behavioral or cognitive neurologist at a memory clinic, not a general neurologist or a psychiatrist. Your gut noticed something real. Your job now is to document it clearly and get it in front of the right person.

Chapter 2. What the FTD Brain Is Doing

Marcus and his wife Jen had been married nineteen years when Jen was diagnosed. They left the neurologist's office with a folder. In the car on the way home, Marcus opened the folder and read the MRI report out loud. "Significant atrophy of the bilateral frontal lobes and anterior temporal poles." He stopped. He looked at Jen, who was scrolling her phone in the passenger seat, humming. He said, "Babe. What does this mean?"

Jen said, "Oh. Yeah. The doctor said my brain is shrinking in those parts."

"Yes, but what does that do?"

Jen shrugged. "He didn't really explain."

Marcus drove home in silence. That night, after Jen fell asleep on the couch at 7:30, he opened his laptop and started reading. He read for six hours. He drank three cups of coffee. At 2 a.m., he wrote down a sentence in his notebook in block letters: "THE BRAIN IS NOT A COMPUTER. IT IS A BUILDING WITH DIFFERENT ROOMS. SOME OF HER ROOMS ARE COLLAPSING."

The next morning, he had a framework. He understood, for the first time, why Jen had stopped laughing at his jokes, why she would eat an entire sleeve of Oreos without offering him one, why she had started telling their teenage son his acne looked bad, why she had not cried at her own father's funeral. It was not a new personality. It was the disappearance of specific old ones, one at a time, as specific parts of her brain stopped working.

Understanding your partner's brain will not save them. It will not slow the disease. What it will do is give you a structure to hang your days on. It will turn confusion into explanation. It will let you say, with accuracy and without blame, "that is the orbitofrontal cortex," rather than, with grief and rage, "that is a stranger I used to love."

Chapter Principle

FTD is not one disease. It is a family of diseases that share the same battlefield, the frontal and anterior temporal lobes. Different regions degenerate in different people, which produces dramatically different clinical pictures. Knowing which regions are involved in your partner's case is not academic. It is the single most useful piece of information you can carry into every day that follows.

2.1 Frontal and Temporal Lobes Do What

The frontal lobes are the part of the brain that sits behind the forehead. If you put your palms on your forehead right now, you are covering them. They are the last part of the brain to mature in humans, finishing development in the mid-twenties, and they are the part of the brain that separates us from most other animals in terms of social behavior.

The frontal lobes run the functions you probably take for granted as "being a person." They run planning and judgment, meaning the capacity to think through consequences before acting. They run social filter, meaning the internal voice that says "do not say that out loud." They run empathy, meaning the capacity to recognize and respond to another person's emotional state. They run motivation, meaning the capacity to get up and do something. They run self-reflection, meaning the capacity to watch yourself and judge your own behavior.

When the frontal lobes shrink, those functions go. Planning goes first in many cases, which is why the person starts to seem scattered at work or unable to manage projects they used to run smoothly. Social filter goes, which is why they start saying things in public they would never have said before. Empathy goes, which is the most devastating loss, because it is the thing that makes your partner feel like your partner. Motivation goes, which looks like laziness or depression but is neither. Self-reflection goes, which is why they cannot see that anything is wrong.

The anterior temporal lobes, which sit on the sides of the head, just above the ears, run a different set of functions. They run the meaning of words, meaning the capacity to know that "spatula" is a kitchen tool used for flipping things, not just a sound you can produce. They run knowledge of objects and concepts. They run recognition of familiar faces and voices.

When the anterior temporal lobes shrink, language goes in a particular way. Your partner does not forget sentences the way an Alzheimer's patient does. They lose the meaning of individual words, one at a time. "Spatula" becomes a sound that does not connect to anything. Then "whisk." Then "pan." Eventually "kitchen." The sentences stay grammatical. The vocabulary just hollows out.

2.2 Why FTD Is Not Alzheimer's

Almost every family member you talk to will call what your partner has "Alzheimer's." They will be wrong, and you will have to decide, over and over, how much energy to spend correcting them.

Alzheimer's is primarily a memory disease. It starts in the hippocampus, which sits deep in the middle of the brain and is responsible for forming new memories. The first symptom is usually forgetting recent events. Long-term personality stays mostly intact in the early years. Judgment, empathy, and social filter stay mostly intact.

FTD is primarily a personality and language disease. It starts in the front of the brain, nowhere near the hippocampus. The first symptoms are usually behavioral or linguistic. Memory, in fact, is often relatively preserved for the first several years, which is one of the reasons the disease is missed. Your wife can still remember her mother's birthday and the name of the first boy she kissed. She just cannot stop buying cordless drills (Bang et al., 2015).

The other critical difference is age. Alzheimer's typically strikes after 65, and increases sharply with age. FTD typically strikes between 45 and 65, with a mean onset around 58. When you hear about someone getting a dementia diagnosis in their forties or fifties, it is statistically more likely to be FTD than Alzheimer's.

The practical implication is that the advice you get from people who have been through Alzheimer's may not apply. The support groups you find online may not apply. The memory care facilities that specialize in Alzheimer's may not be well-suited to FTD. The hospice criteria are calibrated for Alzheimer's and can fail you when your partner reaches end stage. We will return to each of these throughout the book.

2.3 The Three Faces of FTD

FTD is not one clinical picture. It is three, sometimes overlapping.

The first is **behavioral variant FTD (bvFTD)**. This is the classic presentation, the one most associated with the word "FTD." The person develops changes in personality, judgment, and social behavior. They become disinhibited, apathetic, or both. They lose empathy. They develop compulsive behaviors. They may develop unusual eating patterns, often a specific craving for sweets and carbohydrates. Memory and language are relatively preserved in the early stages (Rascovsky et al., 2011).

The second is **primary progressive aphasia (PPA)**. This is a language-led version. The person's speech changes first, and personality changes come later if at all. PPA has three subtypes, which matter enormously for day-to-day life:

Semantic variant PPA (svPPA) involves loss of word meaning. The person can speak fluently but cannot remember what words mean. They may ask, looking at a photo of their own mother, "who is that?" The speech is grammatical but vague. This is associated with damage to the anterior temporal lobes.

Nonfluent/agrammatic variant PPA (nfvPPA) involves effortful, broken speech. The person knows what they want to say but cannot get the words out smoothly. Sentences become short, ungrammatical, halting. Grammar collapses. This is associated with damage to the left inferior frontal gyrus, the region Broca identified over a century ago.

Logopenic variant PPA (lvPPA) involves word-finding pauses and difficulty repeating sentences. The person hunts for common words. Often this variant is driven by Alzheimer's pathology rather than the frontotemporal pathologies, which means its trajectory can look a little different (Gorno-Tempini et al., 2011).

The third face of FTD involves **motor symptoms**. FTD can overlap with amyotrophic lateral sclerosis (ALS), producing FTD-ALS, where muscle weakness and wasting appear alongside behavioral or language changes. It can overlap with progressive supranuclear palsy (PSP), producing stiffness, falls, and eye movement problems. It can overlap with corticobasal syndrome (CBS), producing limb rigidity and apraxia. These combined presentations are uncommon but important to recognize because they change the prognosis and the care plan.

Your partner probably has one dominant presentation. As the disease progresses, features from the others may appear. Knowing where you started is the best predictor of where the next year or two will go.

2.4 Proteins, Genes, and What Causes It

FTD is caused by the buildup of specific proteins in specific brain cells. In most cases, the protein is either tau or TDP-43. A smaller number of cases involve a protein called FUS. These proteins clump together, gum up the cell's machinery, and eventually kill the cell. Over years, enough cells die that the affected part of the brain visibly shrinks on an MRI.

Why the proteins clump is the question everyone is trying to answer. In roughly 30 to 40 percent of cases, there is a known genetic cause. The most common genes involved are *C9orf72*, *MAPT*, and *GRN*. If your partner has a family history of early dementia, ALS, or psychiatric disease (particularly bipolar disorder, which can be an early manifestation of *C9orf72*-linked FTD), genetic testing may be relevant. If your partner is the first in their family with any neurological disease, the case is more likely sporadic.

Genetic testing is a decision worth making carefully, and we will return to it in Chapter 3. For now, what you need to know is that the question "is this genetic?" has practical implications for your children and for your partner's siblings, and it deserves a genetic counselor, not a Google search.

Action Challenge

If you do not already know which FTD presentation your partner has, write it down somewhere visible before you finish this chapter. If you do not know, put a note in your phone to ask at the next appointment. The subtype shapes everything that follows, and you will be asked the question a hundred times over the coming years.

2.5 What a Neurologist Will and Will Not Tell You

A neurologist will tell you the diagnosis, the presumed subtype, the imaging findings, and the general prognosis. Most neurologists will not tell you what your life is about to look like. This is not because they do not care. It is because they see you for forty minutes a year and the disease has no reliable timeline.

Expect your neurologist to tell you roughly what the next six months to a year may look like. Expect them to be reluctant to predict beyond that. Average life expectancy from symptom onset is typically cited as eight to ten years, but individual variation is enormous. Some people progress over three years. Some over twenty. FTD-ALS progresses the fastest, often within two to three years. Pure bvFTD can stretch far longer.

What your neurologist will not tell you, because they are not equipped to, is how to explain this to your children, how to handle the in-laws, how to decide when to stop working, how to manage the marriage itself. For those questions, you will build a different team: a behavioral neurology nurse navigator, if your clinic has one, a social worker, a therapist familiar with ambiguous loss, eventually a geriatric care manager, a speech-language pathologist if your partner has PPA, and an attorney. We build that team in Chapters 7 and 12.

From the Person with FTD's Perspective

Neuroscience research on bvFTD suggests that many people with the disease do not experience their own behavioral changes as changes. The internal sense is of acting naturally, as they always have, while the world around them inexplicably reacts poorly. This is the anosognosia described earlier.

For people with PPA, the experience is different. Many people with PPA retain insight well into the disease. They know they cannot find the word. They feel the sentence collapsing in real time. They experience the shrinking of their own language from the inside. Clinicians who work with PPA patients often describe it as the most cruel of the FTD subtypes, because the person is aware of what they are losing.

If your partner has PPA and appears frustrated or withdrawn, it is worth knowing that they may be mourning their own language in real time. Silence is not necessarily disengagement. It may be preserving dignity.

From the Supporting Partner's Perspective

Learning the neuroscience helps more than you expect, and less than you hoped. It helps because it gives you a framework. It lets you say "that's the orbitofrontal cortex" instead of "that's a stranger I used to love." It lets you treat outbursts as symptoms rather than attacks.

It does not help because understanding what is happening in the brain does not change what is happening in your kitchen. Your husband still ate the whole pie. Your wife still insulted your sister. The cortex explanation is true and it is not enough. The grief keeps coming anyway.

Give yourself both. Learn the biology, because it will protect you on the worst days. And do not expect it to protect you on all of them.

Practical Strategies and Scripts

When a relative calls it Alzheimer's: "It's actually called frontotemporal dementia. It's different from Alzheimer's. Memory isn't the main thing. The main thing is personality and behavior." Say it once. Let it go.

When explaining the diagnosis to a doctor who has never seen FTD: "My partner has [bvFTD / svPPA / nfvPPA / lvPPA]. The main features are [behavioral disinhibition / word-meaning loss / effortful speech / word-finding difficulty]. They are cognitively [preserved / affected] in terms of memory. I can send you an AFTD provider info sheet." Bring the sheet to appointments.

When googling for information and getting overwhelmed: Use the AFTD website (theaftd.org), the UCSF Memory and Aging Center website, and the Rare Dementia Support website (raredementiasupport.org) as your first three sources. Avoid forums for the first month. They are invaluable later and crushing early on.

Reflection Prompts

What part of the brain explanation, if any, landed for you? What did it reframe?

What were you calling the changes before you had the FTD framework? What did you call them in your head?

What do you wish your partner's doctor had explained and did not?

Which subtype do you think your partner has? If you are uncertain, where can you get that clarified?

The Quick Version

FTD is a family of diseases that affect the frontal lobes, the anterior temporal lobes, or both. There are three clinical presentations: behavioral variant (bvFTD), primary progressive aphasia (PPA) in three subtypes, and FTD with motor features. Memory is relatively preserved in most FTD subtypes, which is why it is commonly misdiagnosed. About 30 to 40 percent of cases are genetic. Life expectancy from symptom onset varies hugely. Knowing your partner's specific subtype will save you enormous effort and misdirected advice. Your neurologist will tell you the medicine. The rest of the team is something you will have to build yourself.

Chapter 3. The Day Everything Changes

The neurologist had a gentle voice. Priya noticed that first. She noticed the voice before she noticed the words.

The words were: "What we're seeing on imaging, combined with the cognitive testing, is consistent with a form of frontotemporal dementia. Specifically, we think this is the behavioral variant."

Priya's husband Arjun, sitting beside her in the fabric chair, said, "Okay." He said it the way he might have said okay to a parking ticket.

The neurologist asked if they had questions. Priya opened her mouth and found that her mouth had stopped working. She looked at her lap. The neurologist waited. After a long time, Priya said, "How long?"

The neurologist said, "It varies. I don't give ranges because they tend to be wrong."

Priya asked two more questions. She does not remember what they were. The neurologist handed her a pamphlet and told them to make a follow-up appointment in three months.

In the parking garage, Priya could not find the car. She walked up and down level three for ten minutes while Arjun followed her patiently. When she finally found it, she sat in the driver's seat and cried for forty-five minutes. Arjun watched her. He did not cry. He did not ask her why she was crying. He looked at his phone and said, "Are we going home?"

If you have had a day like Priya's, or you are about to have one, this chapter is a map for the first seventy-two hours and the first month. It is not a map for how to feel. You will feel however you feel. It is a map for what to do with your hands.

Chapter Principle

The diagnosis day is the day your life is renamed. Nothing about the disease has changed in the hour since you walked into the office. What changed is the word you are allowed to use for it. The next seventy-two hours are not about processing. They are about pausing. Almost every major decision partners make in the first month they later regret.

3.1 Why the Diagnosis Day Feels Like Amputation

The diagnosis day is its own kind of trauma. It is not the worst day. The worst days come later. But it is the day a door closes behind you that you cannot open again.

Many partners describe the same set of sensations afterward: the parking lot disorientation, the inability to remember what was said, the feeling of being underwater, the fury at the neurologist for not doing more, the fury at the pamphlet for existing, the urge to call everyone and tell no one, the guilt of feeling relieved that someone finally named it, the guilt of feeling relieved that it is your partner and not you (Heming Willis, 2025).

All of this is normal. None of it means you are broken. You have just been told that the person you love has a terminal disease of the brain, on a weekday, in the middle of the afternoon, and then been asked to drive home. The disorientation is not a failure. It is a normal human response to an abnormal human event.

What partners often get wrong in the first few days is trying to think. You cannot think right now. The part of your brain that makes decisions is flooded with the same chemicals that flood a soldier after an ambush. What you can do right now is survive the next few hours. That is enough.

3.2 The Questions to Ask in the Next Appointment

At the first follow-up, ideally within a week or two of the diagnosis, bring a written list of questions. You will not remember them otherwise. Here is a starter set.

What FTD subtype, specifically, are we dealing with? If the neurologist was hedging at the diagnosis appointment, push for more specificity now.

Is there any indication this is genetic? Should we consider genetic counseling? If yes, who do you recommend?

What other specialists should we be seeing? (Expect some combination of: behavioral neurologist, neuropsychologist, speech-language pathologist if PPA, social worker, genetic counselor if indicated, palliative care consult. Yes, palliative care, even early. Their job is not only end-of-life care.)

What research studies are enrolling that my partner might qualify for? (This matters even if you are not sure you want to enroll. Study enrollment sometimes provides access to experts and close monitoring you cannot otherwise get.)

What should we be doing legally and financially right now? (A good neurologist will tell you: power of attorney, soon.)

What behaviors should I watch for that would mean we need to see you sooner than the next scheduled appointment?

Is there a nurse navigator or social worker attached to this clinic we can contact between appointments?

What can we expect over the next six months? I understand you can't predict the whole trajectory, but what should we prepare for in the near term?

3.3 Second Opinions and When to Get One

FTD is frequently misdiagnosed and occasionally correctly diagnosed only to be contradicted by a specialist later. It is reasonable, and sometimes wise, to seek a second opinion, particularly if:

Your partner was diagnosed by a general neurologist rather than a behavioral neurologist.

The imaging findings were described as equivocal or did not clearly match the clinical picture.

Your partner is unusually young (under 50).

There is a strong family history that was not fully explored.

You have a persistent sense that the diagnosis does not quite fit.

The specialty centers for FTD in the United States include the UCSF Memory and Aging Center, the University of Pennsylvania Frontotemporal Degeneration Center, the Mayo Clinic, the Massachusetts General Hospital FTD Unit, and the Memory and Alzheimer's Treatment Center at Johns Hopkins, among others. In the UK, the National Hospital for Neurology and Neurosurgery in London and the Cambridge Centre for Frontotemporal Dementia are major centers. Most of these accept referrals from outside their immediate region, and most offer telehealth consultations.

A second opinion is not disrespectful to your current neurologist. It is responsible medicine. A good neurologist will send records without hesitation.

3.4 Genetic Testing and When to Pursue It

The question of genetic testing deserves a genetic counselor, not a decision made in a parking lot.

Genetic testing has real benefits. It can confirm the diagnosis in ambiguous cases. It can help your children and your partner's siblings understand their own risk. It can open doors to clinical trials that are enrolling based on specific genetic variants. It can inform family planning for younger family members.

Genetic testing also has real costs. A positive result can create pressure on adult children to be tested themselves, which raises psychological, insurance, and life-planning questions that take years to work through. Some families decide together not to test. That is a legitimate choice. It is the family's choice, not the doctor's.

Before you make the decision, meet with a certified genetic counselor. They will walk you through what the testing can and cannot tell you, what the turnaround is, how results get communicated to family, and what insurance issues may be at play (in the United States, the Genetic Information Nondiscrimination Act, GINA, offers some but not all protections). Your neurology clinic should be able to refer you. If they cannot, the AFTD Helpline can.

Action Challenge

Before the next appointment, sit down with your partner, if they can still have the conversation, and write out what you both would want to know or not know about genetic risk. If they cannot, write out what you believe they would have wanted if you had asked them a year ago. That document, dated and signed, is worth more than you realize.

3.5 The First Seventy-Two Hours

In the first seventy-two hours after diagnosis, do these things:

Eat. Sleep if you can. Cancel any non-essential commitments for the next week.

Tell one person. Not everyone. One person, whoever you trust most to hold information carefully. That person's job is to listen and to not offer advice.

Write down the diagnosis exactly as it was given to you, including subtype, and put it somewhere you can find it. You will forget. Everyone does.

Schedule the follow-up appointment. Put it in your calendar. Put it in your partner's calendar.

Order any books or resources you want from AFTD. The Emma Heming Willis book, *The Unexpected Journey* (2025), is a good first read for many partners, not because it is a clinical manual but because it models how another partner survived the first year. Pauline Boss's *Loving Someone Who Has Dementia* (2011) is worth buying now and reading later, when you can.

Do not: call every family member. Post on social media. Quit your job. Put the house on the market. Sign any new financial documents. Make any major life decisions. Have the big conversation with the children yet, unless they already witnessed the appointment.

The first seventy-two hours are about triage, not strategy. The strategy comes in the following weeks.

One more thing, often overlooked: go outside at some point in the first seventy-two hours. Sit on a porch. Walk around the block. Buy a coffee somewhere that does not know your news. Your body has been through a shock, and bodies recover from shocks better in moving air than in closed rooms. This is not a wellness ritual. This is basic nervous system reset. Fifteen minutes outdoors changes your baseline more than most people expect.

3.6 What Not to Do in the First Month

In the first month, many partners make decisions they later unmake at great cost. The most common are:

Selling the house. Many partners feel an urgent need to "simplify" or "downsize." Stay put. The house is familiar to your partner, and familiar environments reduce behavioral symptoms. Sell later, if at all.

Quitting your job. Your income and your insurance matter more now than they did yesterday, not less. You have time to think about work decisions. Do not quit in week two.

Making announcements on social media. Your partner's reputation, employment, and privacy are all still theirs to protect. An announcement cannot be unmade. If you want to tell people, tell people individually.

Having the big conversation with adult children over the phone. If you have children old enough to understand, most family therapists recommend telling them in person when you can. A phone call breaks the news. A visit holds it.

Starting arguments with siblings over who will help. You are not ready to negotiate this. Your siblings and in-laws are not ready to negotiate this. Give it a month.

Making medical decisions in anger at the system. If you leave the diagnosis appointment angry at the neurologist, do not fire them in week two. You may need them later. Decide when you are not flooded.

Committing to a specific care plan. Partners sometimes announce, in the first two weeks, a firm plan for the next five years: we will stay in this house, we will never use memory care, we will handle everything at home, or the opposite, we will move to be near our daughter next month. Almost none of these announcements survive contact with the actual disease. Hold the plans loosely. You will learn more in month six than you could have known in week two.

From the Person with FTD's Perspective

On diagnosis day, many people with bvFTD show minimal reaction. This is not denial. It is the neurological loss of insight, combined with reduced emotional responsiveness that is itself a feature of the disease. Your partner may not grieve the diagnosis the way you expect. This does not mean they do not understand in some way. It means the parts of their brain that would have produced that grief are no longer producing it.

For people with PPA, the reaction is often different. Many PPA patients cry on the diagnosis day. They understand. They have feared this for months. Their reaction may be closer to yours.

Either response is the disease, not the person. Do not read too much into what they did or did not show in the office. You will have years to learn what they still feel and how they still express it.

From the Supporting Partner's Perspective

The diagnosis day will become a date you remember for the rest of your life. You will remember what you were wearing. You will remember the parking garage. You will remember the exact words the neurologist used. You will not remember what you were supposed to do on Tuesday.

For the first few weeks, you may find yourself functioning at about sixty percent of your usual capacity. This is a normal stress response. Lower your standards accordingly. Cook simpler meals. Respond to fewer emails. Say no to things. Your job right now is to keep yourself and your partner intact for the next appointment.

You have not failed anything. You have just been handed a life you did not order.

Practical Strategies and Scripts

When people ask how you are in the first week: "We got some hard news. I'm not up to talking about it yet. Thank you for asking." End of script. You do not owe anyone a diagnosis disclosure on their timeline.

When someone offers unsolicited advice in the first week: "Thank you. I'm not at a point where I can absorb suggestions yet. I'll come back to you when I am." Repeat as needed.

When your partner seems unaffected by the diagnosis: Do not try to make them feel something. The absence of response is a symptom. Love them through the flatness. Do not argue with it.

When you cannot stop crying: Set a timer for fifteen minutes. Cry. When the timer goes off, drink a glass of water and do one concrete thing, even if it is folding laundry. The timer will not stop the grief. It will give the grief a container so you can also function.

Reflection Prompts

What did you do in the first seventy-two hours after the diagnosis? What would you tell someone else to do?

Is there a decision you feel pressure to make right now? What happens if you delay it thirty days?

Who is the one person you have told, or would tell, first? Why that person?

What do you wish the neurologist had said that they did not?

The Quick Version

The diagnosis day renames everything but changes nothing about the disease itself. The next seventy-two hours should be triage: eat, sleep, tell one person, schedule the follow-up, order resources. The first month should avoid major life decisions, which are almost always regretted. A second opinion at an FTD specialty center is reasonable, especially for younger patients or ambiguous cases. Genetic testing deserves a genetic counselor, not a parking-lot decision. Your partner's reaction on diagnosis day is the disease showing itself, not a window into how they really feel.

Chapter 4. Not Them But the Disease

Raúl had been furious at his wife for eight months.

He had not told anyone. He was ashamed. Elena had been diagnosed with bvFTD a year earlier, and Raúl had read everything he could find, and he still, every single day, could not stop being furious at her. She had made their son cry at Thanksgiving. She had laughed during a condolence call for his cousin's dead baby. She had stopped saying "I love you" back. She had spent $4,000 on a guitar she did not know how to play and left it in the garage.

He knew, intellectually, that these were symptoms. He knew the word "symptom." He knew which part of her brain was shrinking. He had the AFTD folder. He had the pamphlets.

None of it helped. When she said something cruel, he went stiff. When she did not say "I love you" back, he had to leave the room. When he saw the guitar in the garage, he thought, with a clarity that horrified him, *I hate her*.

Eight months in, at his first support group on a Tuesday night in a church basement, Raúl finally said it out loud. He said, "I know she has a disease. I still hate her every day."

The woman facilitating the group, whose husband had died of bvFTD four years earlier, did not flinch. She said, "Of course you do. She is destroying the person you married. The fact that it is not her fault does not make it hurt less."

Raúl put his face in his hands. The woman said, quietly, "The hate is grief in a costume. It is still grief. Let yourself have it."

He cried for the first time since the diagnosis.

This chapter is about the single most important reframe you will make about your partner. It is not a reframe that comes easily, and it is not a reframe that eliminates the hardest feelings. It is a reframe that lets you keep loving them, and keep yourself, when everything else in the relationship is changing faster than you can track.

Chapter Principle

The behaviors that hurt you are not coming from the person. They are coming from specific damaged brain regions that the person cannot override. Understanding this does not stop the hurt. It redirects the anger. It is the difference between being at war with your spouse and being at war with a disease your spouse also cannot control.

4.1 The Brain Is Not Choosing This

The human brain contains about 86 billion neurons. The frontal lobes, the part affected first in bvFTD, contain roughly 20 percent of them. When those neurons die, the functions they performed do not get rerouted. They disappear.

This is not like a muscle that can be retrained. This is not like a habit that can be broken with willpower. This is like the electrical wiring in a house being cut. The light that used to turn on when you flipped the switch no longer turns on, because the wire that carried the signal is gone. You can flip the switch a thousand times. You can shout at the switch. The light is not coming back until you rewire the house, which, in the case of your partner's brain, is not currently possible.

Your partner is not choosing to be cruel. They are not choosing to be apathetic. They are not choosing to spend money you do not have. The choice-making machinery in their brain is breaking down, and the behaviors you are watching are what happens when choice-making breaks down in a human.

This is the hardest thing to hold. It is hardest because the behaviors look like choices. They look exactly like choices. Your partner has a face, and the face makes expressions, and the expressions look like the expressions of someone choosing. The voice sounds like their voice. The words sound like words someone chose to say.

But the structures in the brain that would have generated the choice, that would have paused before the action, that would have considered the consequences, are not working. The output looks like choice. The process behind it is not choice.

4.2 Disinhibition Explained at the Neural Level

Take disinhibition, the symptom that causes most public embarrassment in bvFTD. Disinhibition is the loss of the brain's brake system. The region responsible for this brake system is the orbitofrontal cortex, the part of the frontal lobes that sits just above the eye sockets.

In a healthy brain, when an impulse arises, to say something, to grab something, to touch something, the orbitofrontal cortex checks that impulse against social context, consequences, and personal values, and usually suppresses the impulse. You think about telling your boss she has food in her teeth. The orbitofrontal cortex says, "not like that," and suppresses the impulse. You find another way, or you let it go.

In bvFTD, the orbitofrontal cortex shrinks. The brake stops working. The impulse that would have been suppressed now goes straight through to action. Your partner thinks, "that woman's dress is too tight," and says it, out loud, to the woman, at the grocery store. The impulse was not bigger than usual. The brake that would have stopped it is gone. Clinically, this pattern of socially inappropriate behavior in bvFTD has been described as a form of acquired sociopathy, tied to orbitofrontal damage rather than to the person's premorbid character (Mendez et al., 2005).

When you understand this at the neural level, the behavior stops looking like willful rudeness and starts looking like what it is: the exposed wiring of a human brain without its filter. Your partner is not choosing to be crude. Your partner has lost the part of the brain that would choose not to be.

4.3 Why Loss of Empathy Is Not Loss of Love

Of all the changes in FTD, loss of empathy is the most devastating, because it is the one that feels like a withdrawal of love. The research, though, suggests something more specific and, in a strange way, more bearable.

Research on empathy in bvFTD has shown deficits across both perspective-taking (the cognitive component of empathy) and empathic concern (the emotional component), with these deficits linked to atrophy in right frontal and temporal regions (Rankin et al., 2006). Related work has shown that the loss of warm, agreeable interpersonal traits in neurodegenerative disease is also tied to right-sided frontotemporal atrophy (Sollberger et al., 2009). Even so, partners often report that warmth, attachment, and the capacity for affection persist in different forms; what is most visibly lost is the moment-to-moment ability to read your face, recognize your distress, and respond to it.

This matters because it changes how you interpret the absence. Your partner does not comfort you when you cry because they cannot read "crying" as distress requiring response. This is not because they have stopped loving you. It is because the circuitry that would have translated their love into caregiving behavior is damaged. The love may still be there. The expression of it has lost its engine.

Many long-term partners of people with FTD describe moments, years into the disease, when their person reaches for them in bed at night, or smiles at a familiar song, or squeezes their hand without being asked. These moments are evidence that something underneath the surface has not disappeared. What is gone is the translation layer, not necessarily the underlying feeling.

This framing does not make the absence of comfort easier. It does give you a way to stop reading the absence as a verdict on your relationship.

4.4 When Anger at Them Is Actually Anger at the Disease

Raúl's breakthrough in the church basement was not the discovery that his wife was sick. He knew that. His breakthrough was the recognition that the fury he felt every day was not actually at her. It was at the disease. But the disease does not have a face, and she does.

This is one of the cruelest tricks of loving someone with FTD. The entity destroying your life lives inside the body of the person you love. There is nowhere else for your anger to land. Your anger has to go somewhere, and the only available target is wearing their face, eating their breakfast, sleeping in your bed.

Recognizing this does not make the anger go away. It does let you, over time, begin to aim it differently. You can be furious at the disease while still being tender with the person. You can punch a pillow. You can scream in the car. You can cry in a support group that the facilitator's husband is dead and that some days you wish the same for your wife so the waiting would be over, and you can know, the next morning, that this does not mean you do not love her. It means you are exhausted, and the disease is cruel, and humans under chronic cruelty sometimes wish for the cruelty to end.

The goal is not to stop being angry. The goal is to stop spending the anger on the person who cannot defend themselves against it, because they did not choose it, and because they cannot recover from it being directed at them. Aim the anger at the disease. Aim it at the medical system. Aim it at the pharmaceutical companies who have not yet produced a treatment. Aim it at the inadequate insurance. Aim it at the friends who disappeared. Aim it anywhere except the human who is as much a victim of this as you are.

Action Challenge

For the next week, when you notice anger rising at your partner, silently name the brain region responsible for the behavior. "That is her orbitofrontal cortex." "That is his anterior temporal lobe losing the word." Do this even if it feels forced. Many partners report a measurable shift in reactivity within days. You are not trying to stop feeling angry. You are trying to stop aiming it at the person.

4.5 The Reframe That Keeps You From Drowning

Partners who survive the long arc of FTD tend to describe, in one form or another, the same reframe. It is the reframe Raúl found in the church basement. It is the reframe Linda found after the neurologist finally said "frontotemporal" out loud. It is the reframe Priya found six months after the diagnosis, when she stopped expecting Arjun to ask her how her day was.

The reframe is this: my partner and I are now on the same side of a disease we are both living with. The disease is the opponent. We are the team.

This is not a sentimental framing. It is a structural one. Before the reframe, you are two people trapped in a failing marriage. After the reframe, you are two people fighting a disease that happens to be eating one of you. The person with FTD is not the adversary. The disease is.

This does not mean your partner stops causing pain. They will. It does not mean you stop feeling lonely. You will, often. It does not mean the grief goes away. It will last the rest of your life in some form.

What the reframe does is give you somewhere to stand. When your partner does something that would have been, before the disease, an act of cruelty or betrayal, you can step back and ask: is this them, or is this the disease? Most of the time, the answer is the disease. And then the question becomes: how do I, on behalf of both of us, handle this?

That is the question this whole book is trying to help you answer.

From the Person with FTD's Perspective

Most people with bvFTD cannot articulate what it is like to be them. They do not have access to the self-reflection that would be required. Brief glimpses sometimes emerge, particularly in early disease or during unexpected lucid moments. In these glimpses, people occasionally describe a sense of the world being somehow blunted, less compelling, less sharp. They do not describe feeling cruel. They describe feeling, if anything, normal.

For people with PPA, where insight is often preserved longer, the experience is frequently of frustration at the mismatch between intention and output. They intend to say something kind. Something else comes out, or nothing comes out, or what comes out does not match what they meant. The distance between meaning and saying widens.

Your partner is not choosing the behaviors. In most cases, they are also not aware of choosing them or not choosing them. The behaviors are emerging from a brain whose architecture is shifting, and the self that would have chosen is shifting along with it.

From the Supporting Partner's Perspective

You will have days when the neuroscience does not help. You will have days when you do not care that it is the orbitofrontal cortex. You will have days when you want, for a moment, to hold your partner responsible for their cruelty, because holding a disease responsible is thin comfort when you are the one bleeding.

Those days are not failures. They are the cost of staying present to a slow loss. You are allowed to have them. You are also allowed to come back to the reframe the next morning, because the reframe is what protects both of you in the long run.

Raúl, two years after the church basement, described it this way: "The hate never fully went away. It comes back sometimes, usually when I'm tired. What changed is that I know now what to do with it. I write it down. I tell my support group. I go for a walk. Then I come back and I feed her dinner. The hate is a weather. The love is the climate."

Practical Strategies and Scripts

When a family member blames your partner for a behavior: "That's not him. That's the disease. He would be horrified if he had the insight to see it. I need you to see it the same way."

When you catch yourself about to say something you will regret to your partner: Leave the room. Close a door. Count to ten. Come back when you are not flooded. Do this as many times as you need. You are not obligated to engage in real time.

When your partner does something cruel and you cannot stop thinking about it: Write it down in a document that is only for you. Describe it in detail. Name the brain region responsible. Close the document. The act of externalizing it, combined with naming the neurology, reduces the grip it has on you.

When you feel anger at the disease but have no outlet: Donate to FTD research, even five dollars. Volunteer a virtual hour for AFTD. Write the advocacy email to your senator about early-onset dementia funding. Directed rage is less corrosive than trapped rage.

Reflection Prompts

What is a behavior your partner has shown that you have been blaming on them rather than on the disease? What would change if you redirected that?

Who in your life still blames your partner? What would it take to educate them, or to stop expecting them to understand?

When you are angry at your partner, what is the anger actually about? Follow it down one layer.

What is one thing your partner still does that shows the love is underneath, even when the expression has changed?

The Quick Version

The behaviors that hurt you are produced by specific damaged brain regions your partner cannot override. Disinhibition, apathy, loss of empathy, compulsive behaviors: each maps to a specific area of brain tissue that is no longer functioning. Understanding this does not eliminate the hurt, but it redirects the anger toward the disease and away from the person. Loss of cognitive empathy is not loss of love; the translation layer breaks down before the underlying attachment does. Partners who survive the long arc of FTD describe the same reframe: my partner and I are on the same side of a disease we are both living with.

PART TWO: THE DAILY REALITY

Part Two is about the work of living. The behaviors, the language changes, the money, the safety. These four chapters cover what most partner books skip: the concrete mechanics of what to do when your husband eats a whole pie, when your wife cannot find the word for spoon, when someone transfers your retirement savings to a stranger on Instagram, when your partner walks out of the house at 5 a.m. and does not come back.

Part One was about understanding. Part Two is about action. Nothing in these four chapters is about how to feel. That is Part Three. These chapters are about what to do, in what order, and what to have ready for the next crisis before it arrives.

Read these with a pen. Most of them have checklists you will want to use.

Chapter 5. Living With Personality Changes

Delia bought the first lockbox on a Tuesday. She cried the whole time she was installing it on the pantry door.

Her husband Thomas, seventy-one, had been eating. She did not know how else to put it. He ate. Constantly. A jar of peanut butter in an afternoon. A family-sized bag of potato chips between lunch and dinner. An entire gallon of ice cream on a Saturday when she had gone to the grocery store for two hours. He had gained thirty-two pounds in four months. His blood sugar was becoming a problem. His knees were becoming a problem.

She had tried reasoning. "Honey, we talked about this. The doctor said." Thomas would nod, say okay, and eat a sleeve of Oreos thirty minutes later, with no apparent memory of the conversation.

She had tried hiding food. Thomas found it. Thomas could find food the way a bloodhound finds fugitives.

She had tried small plates, portion control, healthy alternatives. The small plates just meant he ate six of them.

The lockbox went on the pantry door. She also put one on the refrigerator. She put one on a cabinet with crackers. She felt, installing them, that she was treating her husband like a child, and that it was a kind of failure.

That night she sat at the kitchen table and watched Thomas go to the pantry for his eight o'clock snack. He stood at the locked door for about ninety seconds. He looked confused. Then he turned around, sat on the couch, and watched TV. He did not mention the lockbox. He did not ask about it. He did not seem upset.

Over the next two weeks, Thomas stopped searching for food. He lost five pounds. His mood stabilized. At his next endocrinology appointment, his blood sugar was better than it had been in a year.

Delia cried again, this time in the parking lot of the endocrinology clinic, but for a different reason. She had been interpreting the lockbox as a failure of care. It was, actually, an act of care. The part of Thomas's brain that could stop eating was gone. Her lockbox was a prosthetic for the part that was gone. It was not humiliating him. It was protecting him from a brain that was no longer protecting him.

Chapter Principle

You cannot reason with a damaged frontal lobe. You can only reshape the room around it. This chapter is about the specific behavioral strategies that work in FTD. They will feel, at first, like you are treating your partner like a child. You are not. You are supplying the brain functions they no longer have. That is care, not insult.

5.1 Prevention Always Beats Correction

The fundamental rule of behavioral management in FTD is this: prevention beats correction, every time, without exception.

Correction is what you do after the behavior has happened. "Don't do that." "You can't say that to people." "Remember we talked about this." Correction fails in FTD for a simple reason: the brain region that would have registered the correction and changed the future behavior is the same brain region that is damaged. You are trying to tell the part of your partner's brain that does not work how it should work. It will not take.

Prevention is what you do before the behavior happens. You identify the circumstances that prompt the behavior. You remove the prompt, or you change the environment so the behavior cannot occur, or you redirect your partner before the impulse fires. Prevention works because it does not require anything of the damaged brain. It only requires something of you, the caregiver, and the environment around both of you.

Every strategy in this chapter, and in most of the rest of the book, descends from this principle. Lock the pantry rather than lecture about eating. Drive rather than argue about driving. Move the car keys rather than negotiate about the car keys. Remove the credit card from the wallet rather than discuss spending. The behavior your partner cannot stop is a fact of the disease. Your job is not to convince them to stop. Your job is to make the behavior harder or impossible to perform.

5.2 The ABC Model for Any Behavior

Behavioral specialists working with FTD, autism, and other conditions involving reduced behavioral flexibility use a framework called the ABC model. It stands for Antecedent, Behavior, Consequence. The model is deceptively simple and, once you start using it, will change how you see every difficult day.

The **antecedent** is what happened just before the behavior. It is the cue, the context, the setup. Your partner got hungry. The refrigerator was unlocked. They walked into the kitchen. The chocolate cake was visible on the counter.

The **behavior** is what your partner did. They ate the whole cake.

The **consequence** is what happened after. You came home. You reacted. Maybe you yelled. Maybe you cried. Maybe you cleaned up. Maybe your partner did not react to any of it.

In FTD, the consequence has limited effect on future behavior, because the brain region that would connect consequence to future action is damaged. So you cannot modify the behavior by modifying the consequence. What you can modify is the antecedent. You can lock the refrigerator. You can not leave cake on the counter. You can plan meals so hunger is less intense at the times your partner tends to raid the kitchen. You can redirect with activity before the impulse.

When a difficult behavior happens, do not ask "how do I punish this?" Ask "what was the antecedent, and how do I prevent it next time?" (O'Connor et al., 2019).

5.3 Managing Compulsive Eating and Food Fixation

Hyperorality, the technical name for the eating changes in FTD, affects a majority of people with bvFTD and some people with PPA. It shows up as increased overall intake, a strong craving specifically for sweets and simple carbohydrates, fixation on specific foods (a "food fad"), and sometimes eating of non-food items (Ikeda et al., 2002).

Practical strategies that work:

Remove visual cues. Counters with food on them are a problem. Clear them. If your partner cannot see the cake, the impulse does not fire as often.

Lock what needs to be locked. Pantries, refrigerators, specific cabinets. Lockboxes from Amazon cost under twenty dollars. They are not permanent. You are not a warden. You are a brain supplement.

Pre-portion meals and snacks. Instead of serving family-style, serve plates. Instead of leaving a bag of chips, put one serving in a bowl. The physical absence of the rest of the bag helps.

Schedule eating. Many people with FTD do better with a predictable schedule of meals and snacks than with free access. Schedule four or five small meals a day at consistent times.

Redirect. If your partner starts searching for food thirty minutes after eating, offer something else to do. A walk. A task. A familiar song. The impulse is short-lived. It passes if the brain is occupied with something else.

Talk to the doctor about medications. Some research suggests SSRIs, particularly sertraline and citalopram, can reduce hyperorality in some patients. The evidence is modest but worth discussing.

5.4 When Apathy Looks Like Laziness

Apathy is the single most damaging symptom to the relationship in bvFTD, and it is almost always misunderstood. Apathy is not depression. Apathy is not laziness. Apathy is not a choice.

Apathy is the neurological loss of the capacity to initiate. Your partner is not refusing to get up. They are not able to generate the "get up" signal. Their brain, specifically the medial frontal and anterior cingulate cortex, used to produce thousands of small motivational impulses a day. Get up. Get dressed. Brush your teeth. Do the dishes. Text your daughter. Most of those impulses have gone silent.

What this looks like from the outside is a person sitting on the couch for six hours. What this feels like from the inside, to the extent we can infer it, is neither boredom nor sadness. It is closer to a kind of flat neutrality. The person is not suffering. They are also not enjoying. They are just... there.

Strategies for apathy:

Limit choices. "What do you want for lunch?" is an impossible question. "Do you want a sandwich or soup?" is easier. "I made you a sandwich, here it is" is often easiest.

Cue concretely. Instead of "time to get dressed," lay out the clothes. Instead of "let's go for a walk," hand over the shoes. The cue to action has to be as close to the action itself as possible.

Use routine as a prosthetic. A fixed daily schedule, with the same sequence of activities, reduces the demand on the damaged initiation system. The routine provides the structure that the brain no longer provides internally.

Accompany. Apathy often lifts when the person is accompanied rather than asked to initiate alone. "Let's go for a walk" works better than "you should get some exercise." "Let's eat" works better than "are you hungry?"

Do not interpret apathy as withdrawal from you. This is essential. Your partner is not ignoring you. They cannot produce the motivation to act. If you take it personally, the relationship suffers for a reason that has nothing to do with you.

Action Challenge

For one week, every time you feel frustrated by your partner "not doing" something, reframe: "the initiation signal is not firing, and my job is to be the initiation signal." Track how it changes your reactivity. Most partners report a significant reduction in conflict within days.

5.5 Handling Disinhibition in Public Places

Disinhibition in public produces some of the most exhausting moments of life with FTD. Your partner comments on a stranger's weight. Your partner stands too close to someone in line. Your partner urinates in a place that is not a bathroom. Your partner makes a sexual comment in a business meeting.

Principles for public settings:

Limit public exposure to what is necessary or manageable. You do not have to take your partner everywhere you used to go together. Some outings become no-go. This is a loss, and it is also common sense.

Choose familiar environments. Your partner behaves more predictably in places they know. The same restaurant, the same park, the same coffee shop. Rotate less.

Use FTD awareness cards. A printed card that says "my companion has frontotemporal dementia, a neurological disease that affects behavior. Please excuse anything that seems inappropriate." You can hand it to a server, a clerk, a police officer. AFTD provides templates.

Scout the exit. Before you sit down, know how you will leave. If the behavior escalates, leave. Do not try to finish the meal.

Do not try to correct in the moment. Removing your partner from the situation is faster and more effective than any conversation.

5.6 Medications That Sometimes Help

Pharmacology in FTD is limited. There is no cure, no disease-modifying treatment, and no medication approved specifically for FTD behavioral symptoms. What does exist is a set of medications borrowed from other conditions that sometimes help, with modest evidence.

Selective serotonin reuptake inhibitors (SSRIs), particularly sertraline and citalopram, have some evidence for reducing disinhibition, compulsive behaviors, and hyperorality. They can also help with irritability and mood. The evidence is mixed, mostly drawn from small open-label studies, and a randomized trial of paroxetine did not show benefit (Tsai & Boxer, 2014).

Trazodone, an older antidepressant, has some evidence for reducing behavioral disturbances, including eating behaviors, at moderate doses.

Atypical antipsychotics, including quetiapine, risperidone, and olanzapine, are sometimes used for severe agitation, aggression, or delusions. These carry significant risks in elderly patients, including increased mortality, and should be used only when behavioral management has been insufficient and under close specialist supervision.

Acetylcholinesterase inhibitors (donepezil, rivastigmine, galantamine) are the mainstays of Alzheimer's treatment. They are generally not effective in FTD and can sometimes worsen behavioral symptoms. Your partner should not be on these unless there is a specific indication.

Memantine is also an Alzheimer's drug, and evidence in FTD is mixed, with some studies suggesting it may actually worsen behavior.

The practical guidance: work with a neurologist or neuropsychiatrist who knows FTD. Do not let a primary care provider prescribe Alzheimer's drugs for FTD without specialist input. Start low, go slow, watch for side effects. Behavioral symptoms in FTD respond better to behavioral interventions than to medications in most cases, and medications should be additive, not primary.

From the Person with FTD's Perspective

What does it feel like to eat a whole pie without being able to stop? The honest answer is that we do not fully know, because most people with bvFTD cannot articulate it after the fact. What limited first-person data exist, from rare cases of preserved insight early in the disease, suggest it is less like temptation and more like automatism.

The hand reaches. The food is eaten. There is no deliberative moment that would feel, from the inside, like choice.

For apathy, the internal experience may be closer to flatness than to sadness. Research on apathy in FTD suggests that the person is not experiencing the boredom or frustration they would be expected to experience. The signal that would motivate the next action simply does not arise. Your partner is not miserable on the couch. They are also not happy. They are in something closer to a neutral idle.

If your partner has PPA, the internal experience is often more distressing, because insight tends to be preserved. Your partner may be aware of compulsive behaviors in themselves and ashamed of them. Treat this awareness with care. A person who knows they did something wrong, and cannot stop doing it, is in a different emotional situation than a person who does not know.

From the Supporting Partner's Perspective

You will feel, often, that you are treating your spouse like a child. You will feel, often, that you have become their parent. You will feel, often, that the person you married is gone.

None of these feelings is wrong. All of them are part of the grief of caregiving. Lockboxes, routines, limited choices, scheduled meals, constant redirection: these are exhausting, and they are also acts of love, and they are sometimes humiliating to both of you.

The partners who survive this phase tend to describe, in retrospect, a decision to stop measuring the caregiving against the marriage they used to have. The measurement stick changes. You are not a bad spouse because you lock the pantry. You are a good caregiver who is also still a spouse. These two roles will braid together for the rest of this arc. You did not fail at marriage. You are adapting to a marriage that is surviving a disease.

Practical Strategies and Scripts

The three lockboxes starter kit: pantry door, refrigerator door, one cabinet for high-risk items (medications, alcohol, valuables). Total cost under sixty dollars. Install in an afternoon.

When your partner asks about a lockbox: "The doctor wants us to watch your eating for your blood sugar. This makes it easier." Repeat the same explanation every time asked. You do not need a new story.

When apathy hits at noon and the day feels wasted: Lower the expectation. A single activity, accompanied, counts as a full day. Do not measure the day against what you would have done pre-diagnosis.

When a family member says "you're too controlling": "I'm providing the brain functions his brain can no longer provide. The pantry lock is a medical device. I welcome your help if you'd like to spend a day managing the eating without it."

Reflection Prompts

What is one behavior you have been trying to correct after the fact? What would prevention look like instead?

Which of the ABC model elements (antecedent, behavior, consequence) have you been focused on? What shifts if you move upstream?

What environmental change have you been resisting out of guilt? What would it free up if you made it this week?

Is apathy being mistaken for rejection in your household? How might you reframe a specific recent moment?

The Quick Version

Prevention always beats correction in FTD, because the brain region that would have responded to correction is damaged. The ABC model (antecedent, behavior, consequence) redirects your attention upstream of the behavior. Compulsive eating responds to visual cue removal, lockboxes, pre-portioned meals, and scheduled eating. Apathy is not depression or laziness; it is the loss of initiation, and it responds to concrete cues, limited choices, and accompaniment. Public disinhibition is managed by reducing exposure, using awareness cards, and removing your partner from the situation without trying to correct. Medications exist but are limited; SSRIs and trazodone have the best evidence for behavioral symptoms, and Alzheimer's drugs should generally be avoided.

Chapter 6. Finding Words That Still Work

Mei-Lin and her husband David had been married thirty-four years when David was diagnosed with semantic variant PPA. He was sixty-one. He had been a commercial airline pilot for twenty-eight years and a private instructor for the last six. He had stopped teaching two years earlier when he could not remember the word for "rudder" in front of a student.

By the time the diagnosis came, David could still speak in long, grammatical sentences. But the sentences had grown vague. He no longer used specific nouns. He said "the thing" and "the place" and "that person." He looked at photos of his grandchildren and said, pleasantly, "Who are these people? They look nice."

Mei-Lin adapted without knowing she was adapting. She stopped asking David open-ended questions. She pointed at objects when she spoke. She held up the coffee cup before she asked if he wanted coffee. She answered her own questions. "You want your blue sweater, right? The blue one. Here you go." David would nod. He would smile. He would say, "Yes, that one, the blue one," even though "blue" no longer meant a color to him.

Three years in, at a speech therapy session, the therapist told Mei-Lin that what she had been doing instinctively was what research calls communication partner training. Mei-Lin cried a little. "I thought I was just talking strangely," she said. The therapist said, "You've been keeping him in the conversation when almost nobody else can."

This chapter is for partners of people with primary progressive aphasia, or for partners of people with any FTD variant who are watching language disappear. It is practical. It will teach you what to do and what to stop doing. It will not bring the words back. It will help you keep talking to each other until the last moment when talking is possible, and then help you keep communicating after.

Chapter Principle

Language loss in PPA is not a failure of effort. Your partner is not being lazy, not being rude, not withholding. Their brain is losing specific language functions, one at a time, and most of what well-meaning people instinctively do to help actually makes it harder. This chapter will teach you what to do instead.

6.1 The Three PPA Variants and What Each One Loses

The three subtypes of primary progressive aphasia break language apart in different places. Knowing which one your partner has changes what you should do.

Semantic variant PPA (svPPA) attacks the meaning of words. Your partner can speak fluently. Sentences are grammatical. What is lost is the meaning of individual nouns and verbs, usually starting with less common words and progressing to more common ones. Early on, your partner asks "what is a wren?" Later, they ask "what is a bird?" Still later, they cannot identify a shoe as distinct from a hat. They may also lose recognition of faces and objects. Reading may be affected in a specific way called surface dyslexia, where your partner can read the letter sounds but cannot retrieve meaning. Speech-language pathologists have developed practical, person-centered communication strategies for semantic dementia that focus on personally relevant vocabulary, picture and gesture support, and partner adjustment (Kindell et al., 2015).

Nonfluent/agrammatic variant PPA (nfvPPA) attacks the production of speech. Your partner struggles to get words out. Speech becomes effortful, halting, and grammatically simplified.

Sentences shorten. Small grammatical words ("the," "is," "of") drop out. Your partner may know exactly what they want to say and be unable to say it. Understanding is relatively preserved, at least early. This is the variant most associated with apraxia of speech, where the motor planning of sounds breaks down.

Logopenic variant PPA (lvPPA) attacks word retrieval and sentence repetition. Your partner hunts for common words. They cannot repeat a sentence you just said. Speech is slower than normal but not effortful in the way nfvPPA is. Grammar and word meaning are relatively preserved early on. This variant is often driven by Alzheimer's pathology rather than frontotemporal pathology, and its trajectory can include memory symptoms earlier than the other PPAs.

Your partner probably has one dominant variant. As the disease progresses, features may overlap. Speech-language pathologists with expertise in PPA can track this over time and recommend adjustments.

6.2 Communication Partner Training Basics

Communication partner training is what speech-language pathologists call the work of teaching the spouse, not the patient, how to communicate more effectively. The most studied program is Better Conversations with PPA (BCPPA), developed in the UK, which has early evidence for improving everyday conversation (Volkmer et al., 2023).

The core principles are simple to state and hard to practice.

Slow down. Your pace, not theirs. Give long pauses. Count to ten silently before filling a silence. Most partners fill silences too fast.

Simplify. One idea per sentence. "We're going to the store. Then we're coming home." Not "I thought we could go to the store and maybe swing by the dry cleaner if you're feeling up to it and then pick up your mother for dinner."

Use concrete nouns and shared context. Point at things. Gesture. Show the object. Speech is only one channel. Use all the others.

Ask yes or no questions when possible. "Do you want coffee?" not "What do you want to drink?" Open-ended questions are exhausting in PPA. Forced-choice questions ("coffee or tea?") are a middle ground.

Wait. If your partner is trying to produce a word, wait. The word may come. If it does not, offer one word at a time as a prompt, not a whole sentence.

Repeat if needed, but do not shout. Louder does not help. Slower and simpler does.

Use writing, drawing, or photos to supplement. A printed grocery list. A picture of the grandchild's new baby. A map of the route. Any non-verbal channel is a gift.

6.3 Rules Partners Break That Make It Worse

There are specific habits that well-meaning partners develop that, according to research and speech-language pathology practice, make PPA conversations harder. Most partners do some or all of these without realizing. Stopping them is a concrete, immediate improvement.

Finishing their sentences. This feels helpful. It is not. It takes the language work away from your partner, who may have been about to produce the word. It also signals that you are impatient, which increases their anxiety, which makes retrieval harder. Let them finish. Wait the full pause.

Correcting pronunciation or word choice. "No, you mean *fork*." This rarely produces learning and frequently produces shame. If the meaning was clear, let it stand. If the meaning was not clear, clarify gently, not by correcting but by confirming: "You want the thing to eat with? Here's a fork."

Quizzing. "What's this?" pointing at a spoon. "Who is this in the picture?" Quizzes are exhausting and, in PPA, often painful. They are a feature of assessment, not a feature of love. Stop quizzing.

Talking about your partner in their presence as if they were not there. Many people with PPA retain much of their comprehension well into the disease, especially in nfvPPA and svPPA. They can hear you tell the doctor how hard it has gotten. They can hear you tell your sister on the phone that he is getting worse. Keep them in the conversation, even when they cannot respond in words.

Volunteering to translate. In social settings, when your partner is struggling to speak, many spouses jump in to translate. Sometimes this is necessary. Often it is not. Give your partner the chance to speak, even haltingly. Your jumping in teaches the social circle to stop trying, and the circle shrinks.

6.4 Tools, Boards, and Technology That Help

As speech becomes more limited, augmentative and alternative communication (AAC) tools become useful. These are low-tech or high-tech ways of supplementing or replacing spoken language.

Photo books and memory books. A simple photo album of family members, favorite places, favorite foods, with names labeled. Your partner can point when they cannot find the word.

Topic boards. Printed pages with common categories (food, people, places, feelings) organized with pictures. Your partner points to the category, then you help narrow down.

AAC apps. Apps like Proloquo2Go, TouchChat, and Lingraphica are designed for aphasia. Some are expensive and some are covered by insurance. A speech-language pathologist can evaluate for AAC and help you choose.

Writing. For some people with nfvPPA and lvPPA, writing is preserved longer than speech. A small notebook or a phone notes app can be a lifeline. Let your partner write rather than speak if writing is easier.

Gesture. Do not underestimate gesture. Many couples develop rich non-verbal signals. A tap on the shoulder, a hand squeeze, a shake of the head. These become your shared language.

Action Challenge

This week, pick one of the partner habits in section 6.3 that you do and stop doing it. Just one. Track the effect over seven days. Most partners notice a change in conversational dynamics within the first few days.

6.5 When They Stop Talking Altogether

Late PPA, in all three subtypes, tends toward muteness. Your partner speaks less and less. Eventually they may stop producing spoken language entirely. This can happen years after diagnosis, and the timeline varies.

Muteness is not the end of communication. Many couples describe the late PPA phase as requiring more communication work, not less. You learn to read micro-expressions. You learn to interpret gestures. You learn what a specific hand squeeze means. You learn what the morning routine looks like when your partner is content versus when they are uncomfortable.

What becomes essential is vigilance about basic needs. A person who cannot speak cannot tell you they are in pain, thirsty, or needing the bathroom. You have to anticipate. Schedule offers: every hour or two, ask "are you thirsty?" even if they cannot answer, and offer water. Offer the bathroom at regular intervals. Watch for signs of discomfort: frowning, restlessness, changes in breathing.

6.6 Connection After Language Is Gone

A neurologist working at the UCSF Memory and Aging Center once said something in a lecture that has stuck with many families. He said: "The patient stops speaking. They do not stop being present. The partners who thrive late are the ones who stop needing the speaking to feel the presence."

Music often reaches past language. A song your partner loved before the disease may still reach them when words cannot. Play it. Watch their face. You will see what you need to see.

Touch reaches past language. Hand on the shoulder. Fingers through the hair. Hand held in the bed. Your partner's nervous system still recognizes your touch, long after the name for your face has gone.

Familiar routine reaches past language. Morning coffee at the same table. Evening walk on the same route. Your partner may not be able to narrate what is happening, but their body knows the shape of the day.

Shared food reaches past language. Not as nutrition. As ritual. Sitting down together. Eating the same thing. The communion of a meal predates speech by hundreds of thousands of years.

Your partner is still there. The language is a medium, not the person. When the medium breaks down, other channels open. You will find them, because you have known this person for decades, and decades of love built more channels than words.

From the Person with FTD's Perspective

For many people with PPA, insight into their own language loss is preserved well into the disease. They know they cannot find the word. They feel the sentence collapsing. They often stop speaking in social settings because the effort is exhausting and the embarrassment is real.

What your partner may need from you most, early and mid-disease, is not help. It is patience. Unhurried attention. The absence of the panicked look on your face when they cannot find a word. When you relax, they relax. When you wait, they can often work their way to the word. When you rush or jump in, the word retreats.

In late disease, when speech is largely gone, some families describe sensing their person is still "in there." Research on this is limited. What is clearer is that late PPA patients continue to respond to familiar voices, familiar music, familiar touch, and to show consistent preferences for favorite foods, places, and people. Whatever else is happening internally, something is. Act as if your partner is listening, because the evidence suggests, in ways we do not fully understand, that they often are.

From the Supporting Partner's Perspective

You will become tired, in a specific way, of being the one who carries the conversation. You will miss, specifically, the sentences your partner used to say. Not all of them. Some of them. The way they answered a specific question. The phrase they used when they were proud of you. The joke they told every Thanksgiving.

The loss of specific sentences is its own grief, separate from the disease as a whole. Let yourself feel it. Write down the sentences you miss, so you do not forget them, because when the language is gone, the memory of what the language sounded like is the next thing the years will come for.

Mei-Lin, three years after the diagnosis, started a document she called "Things David Used to Say." She added to it when she thought of one. It had 218 entries by the end of year four. She did not share it. She just kept it. "It's my backup copy of him," she said.

Practical Strategies and Scripts

In a restaurant, when your partner cannot read the menu: "They have a chicken dish you liked last time. Want me to order that?" You are proposing a familiar option, not quizzing.

When a family member on the phone does not know what to do: Email them a one-page guide. "David has a kind of dementia that affects his language. He can hear you and understand most of what you say. He may not respond in words. Please keep talking to him. Let him know you love him. You can hang up whenever it feels right."

When your partner is struggling to produce a word and you know it: Wait. Count to ten in your head. If still stuck, offer a single word, not the full sentence. "Were you saying... *fork*?" Let them confirm.

When a stranger treats your partner as incompetent: "He understands you. He has a speech condition. You can talk to him directly." Do not over-explain.

Reflection Prompts

Which of the partner habits in 6.3 do you catch yourself doing? Which one do you want to stop first?

What non-verbal channel (music, touch, routine, food) already works well in your relationship? How can you build more of it?

If you started a "Things They Used to Say" document today, what would the first entry be?

What is one thing you still want to say out loud to your partner, while you both still have the language? When will you say it?

The Quick Version

PPA has three subtypes (semantic, nonfluent/agrammatic, and logopenic), and each affects language differently. The most useful intervention is communication partner training: slow down, simplify, use yes/no questions, wait, and supplement with writing, pictures, and gesture. Common partner habits that make conversation harder include finishing sentences, correcting pronunciation, quizzing, and translating unnecessarily. As speech fades, other channels open: music, touch, routine, shared food. Your partner is still present even when language is gone. The medium changes. The person remains.

Chapter 7. Protecting Your Financial Future

Caroline discovered the transfer at 6:47 a.m. on a Saturday.

She was making coffee when she opened the banking app, like she always did, and saw that $22,000 had moved from their joint savings account to an account she did not recognize, the day before, at 4:13 p.m. She put the coffee cup down. She sat on the kitchen floor. She opened her husband Bill's phone, because he was still asleep, and went through his messages.

The messages were to a woman on Instagram who claimed to be a US Army veteran stationed in Syria. She had been messaging Bill for six weeks. She had told him she loved him. She had told him she needed money for a medical procedure for her daughter. She had asked him not to tell his wife because his wife did not understand their connection.

Bill had been diagnosed with bvFTD eleven months earlier. Caroline had taken over the bills. She had cancelled his credit cards. She had, she thought, locked down the finances. She had not thought to monitor his Instagram.

The bank was sympathetic and useless. The money was gone. The FBI tip line said they would add it to a database. The scammer's account was deleted within an hour of Caroline reporting it.

Caroline spent the weekend doing three things. She filed a police report. She contacted a lawyer about power of attorney, which they had been "meaning to get to." And she made a spreadsheet of every account, every card, every password, every login, every retirement fund, every insurance policy, and every online platform Bill had access to. The spreadsheet took her eleven hours to complete. She cried the entire time.

On Monday morning she called a certified financial planner who specialized in families dealing with cognitive impairment. She did not know such a specialty existed. It does. The planner's first sentence was, "Let's make sure this does not happen again." They built a plan over the next six weeks that rebuilt the financial architecture of the marriage from scratch.

Chapter Principle

Mental capacity is a cliff, not a slope. It can be there on Tuesday and gone on Wednesday. The legal and financial work has to happen while it is still there, which is usually sooner than you think. This chapter is the checklist of what to do and in what order. None of it is optional. All of it is urgent.

7.1 Mental Capacity and the Clock You Cannot See

In law and in medicine, "mental capacity" refers to the ability to understand, weigh, and communicate a decision. Capacity is task-specific. Your partner may still have capacity to decide what to eat for lunch and not have capacity to decide if they should sign a mortgage refinance. Capacity can fluctuate day to day. Capacity can be present for simple decisions and absent for complex ones.

In FTD, capacity is typically lost earlier and more unpredictably than in Alzheimer's, because the executive functions involved in weighing options are exactly what the disease attacks first. A person with bvFTD may hold conversations, recognize family, and tell you what they had for breakfast while being entirely incapable of understanding a financial contract.

For any legal document that requires capacity, the bar is this: can your partner understand the nature and consequences of the document at the moment of signing? If they can, the document is valid. If they cannot, the document may be challenged later, and the challenge may succeed.

The practical implication: do the paperwork now. Do not wait until it feels urgent. By the time it feels urgent, your partner may no longer have capacity to sign. You will then be looking at guardianship proceedings, which are expensive, contested, and slow.

7.2 Durable Power of Attorney Done Right

The single most important document to get in place is a durable power of attorney (POA). "Durable" means it remains in effect if the principal (your partner) becomes incapacitated, which is the entire point. Without "durable" language, the POA expires at the moment it becomes most needed.

Two types of POA matter. A **financial POA** lets you manage money, accounts, property, taxes, and contracts on your partner's behalf. A **healthcare POA** (also called a healthcare proxy or medical power of attorney) lets you make medical decisions when your partner cannot.

Both should be prepared by an attorney familiar with elder law or cognitive impairment. Do not download a generic template from the internet. State laws vary. Specific language matters. An attorney-drafted POA that costs $500 now can prevent a $30,000 guardianship proceeding later.

Distribute copies. A POA that lives in your filing cabinet is useless in an emergency. Send copies to your bank, your financial advisor, your partner's healthcare providers, and any other institution where you will need to act on your partner's behalf. Keep digital copies accessible on your phone.

Also important: your partner should name a successor agent in case something happens to you. If you are the primary POA holder and you die first, who takes over? This is not a pleasant question. It is a required one.

7.3 The Social Security Compassionate Allowances Fast Track

Since 2011, all forms of frontotemporal dementia have been on the Social Security Administration's Compassionate Allowances list. This is a program that expedites Social Security Disability Insurance (SSDI) and Supplemental Security Income (SSI) decisions for conditions that obviously meet disability criteria.

For a typical SSDI application, processing takes 6 to 18 months, with most initial applications denied and requiring appeals. For a Compassionate Allowances application, decisions can come in as little as a few weeks, and the approval rate for eligible conditions is dramatically higher.

To access the program:

Apply for SSDI through the Social Security Administration (SSA) website or by phone.

In the application, clearly list the diagnosis as "frontotemporal dementia" (not "dementia" or "cognitive impairment" generically).

When you speak to an SSA representative, say explicitly: "This condition is on the Compassionate Allowances list. I would like this application flagged for expedited review."

Provide documentation from the neurologist, including the formal diagnosis letter, imaging reports, and neuropsychological testing results.

If your partner is under 65 and has been working, SSDI will pay cash benefits and, after 24 months, qualify them for Medicare. If your partner has not worked enough to qualify for SSDI, SSI may be available, which also provides Medicaid access in most states.

This step alone can mean the difference between financial stability and bankruptcy. Do it within the first few months.

7.4 Medicare, Medicaid, and Long-Term Care Reality

American healthcare financing for FTD is a patchwork that frequently fails families. Here is the architecture, simplified.

Medicare (federal, for people 65+ or on SSDI for 24 months) covers hospitalizations, doctor visits, and certain skilled nursing for limited periods. Medicare does not cover long-term custodial care. This is the most misunderstood point in dementia financing. The assisted living facility, the memory care facility, the in-home aide who helps with bathing: Medicare does not pay for these. Many families discover this after a hospitalization, when the discharge planner says "Medicare doesn't cover the next step."

Medicaid (federal-state, for low-income individuals) does cover long-term care, including nursing homes and, in many states, in-home care. To qualify, your partner's income and assets must be below state thresholds, which typically requires spending down assets first. The "Medicaid spend-down" is a major financial planning topic, with rules varying by state. Specialized elder-law attorneys can help structure asset protection within legal limits. Start this conversation at least five years before you anticipate needing Medicaid, because the Medicaid look-back period penalizes certain asset transfers made within five years of application.

Long-term care insurance, if your partner bought a policy before diagnosis, may cover some care costs. Check the policy. Understand the elimination period (how long before benefits start) and the daily benefit. After diagnosis, long-term care insurance is no longer obtainable, which is one of the reasons people buy it young.

VA benefits are available for veterans with FTD, including Aid and Attendance benefits that can help with in-home or facility care costs. If your partner served in the military, contact a Veterans Service Officer (VSO) for a benefits review.

The average cost of memory care in the United States in 2025 is approximately $6,000 to $9,000 per month, depending on region. The Galvin et al. (2017) study cited $120,000 per year as the average full cost of FTD care. These numbers drive financial decisions for the remainder of the arc.

7.5 Protecting Assets From Impulsive Spending

Disinhibition and compulsive behaviors in FTD produce specific financial risks. Studies of financial errors in dementia have found that people with bvFTD are more likely than those with Alzheimer's disease to spend excessively, give money inappropriately, and make impulsive purchases (Chiong et al., 2014). The most common patterns include online shopping binges, romance scams (as Caroline encountered), subscription traps, gambling, and unwise investments pitched to older adults. Protection requires layered defenses.

Freeze credit at all three bureaus. This prevents new accounts being opened in your partner's name. Equifax, Experian, and TransUnion. Free to do, free to lift.

Separate accounts. Move most money to an account that does not have your partner's name on it. Keep a small checking account jointly held for necessary expenses.

Card controls. Many banks and card issuers now offer transaction alerts, spending limits, and specific-merchant blocks. Set alerts on every transaction over a low threshold (e.g., $50). Set daily limits.

Payment card instead of credit card. Consider a prepaid debit card for your partner's discretionary use, with a limited weekly reload. This preserves autonomy within a cap.

Remove PayPal, Venmo, and app-store payment methods from your partner's phone. Disable in-app purchases. Turn on screen time restrictions.

Monitor social media. Scammers target older adults through Facebook and Instagram. Either keep your partner off these platforms or monitor messages regularly. This feels invasive. It is. It is also how you prevent the $22,000 call on a Saturday morning.

Mail management. Redirect mail if possible. Scams frequently arrive by physical mail (fake sweepstakes, unsolicited investment offers). Open your partner's mail.

Action Challenge

Before you finish this chapter, do these three things: freeze credit at all three bureaus (15 minutes each, can be done online), set up transaction alerts on every joint account (10 minutes), and apply for SSDI under Compassionate Allowances if not already done (1 to 2 hours for the initial application).

7.6 Updating Wills, Beneficiaries, and Trusts

While your partner still has capacity, update:

Wills. Both yours and theirs. A will drafted five or ten years ago may not reflect current circumstances. Include specific provisions for what happens if you die first, leaving your partner disabled.

Beneficiaries on retirement accounts and life insurance. These pass outside of probate and override wills. Make sure they are current and that contingent beneficiaries are named.

Trusts. Depending on asset level and state, a revocable living trust may simplify management and protect privacy. A special needs trust or a third-party trust may be appropriate to protect assets for a disabled spouse while preserving Medicaid eligibility.

Digital assets. Passwords, logins, two-factor authentication devices. Document everything. A password manager with emergency access provisions (such as 1Password, LastPass, or Bitwarden) can be invaluable.

Work with an estate attorney who understands disability planning. This is a specialty within estate law. A general estate attorney may not know the Medicaid rules, the trust structures, or the disability-specific considerations.

7.7 What Happens If You Die First

This is the question every care partner avoids and must eventually answer. If you die before your partner, who takes over? Where does your partner live? Who manages the money? Who advocates in medical settings?

Write out a plan. A specific plan. Include:

Who the successor POA is (legal and healthcare).

Where your partner will live (stay in the house with paid caregivers? move to memory care? move in with an adult child?).

Who will manage finances and pay bills.

What the budget looks like and where the money comes from.

What your partner's end-of-life wishes are (more on this in Chapter 15).

Key contacts: neurologist, attorney, financial advisor, insurance policies.

Review this document annually. Share it with the successor POA and at least one other trusted person. This is not morbid. This is responsible.

The care partner who does this work is not predicting their own death. They are protecting their partner from the chaos of improvisation. You are building a system that works even if the central node (you) is removed.

From the Person with FTD's Perspective

Your partner cannot see the financial decay the way you can. The disease blunts their awareness of money, their ability to track consequences, and their judgment about who to trust. They are not making bad financial decisions in the way a mentally intact adult would be. They are operating with equipment that no longer does the math.

In early disease, your partner may still feel they should be managing the money, because that was their role for decades. Removing that role can feel to them like a loss of agency and respect. Frame it as a team change, not a demotion. "The doctor wants us to simplify things so we can focus on you feeling better." The exact words do not matter as much as the tone of we-not-you.

By mid-disease, most people with FTD have little interest in financial details. The transition becomes easier. Your task shifts from negotiating with a reluctant partner to simply running the system on their behalf.

From the Supporting Partner's Perspective

You will feel, at some point, that you are stealing from your own partner. You are not. You are protecting both of you. The signing away of a POA, the locking of accounts, the freezing of credit: these will feel, especially early, like a transgression against a healthy adult who is still sitting across the table from you.

Caroline, three years after the Instagram scam, said this to a group of newly diagnosed couples: "I wish I had not waited to do the paperwork. I waited because it felt like I was admitting he was sick. The paperwork is not a prediction. It is a safety net. You do not wait for the floor to collapse to put up a safety net. You put it up while the floor is still solid."

The financial work, done early, is one of the most loving things you can do for your partner. It protects the resources they will need to live well through this disease. It is not a betrayal. It is the infrastructure of care.

Practical Strategies and Scripts

When you set up a POA and your partner resists: "This is what everyone our age does now. The lawyer recommended it for both of us. It doesn't take anything away from you, it just means if something happens to either of us, the other can keep things running."

When a relative questions your financial moves: "We've put these protections in place with our attorney and financial planner. I'm happy to share the general structure if it's helpful. I'm not looking for feedback on the specifics." Firm. Polite. No explanation owed.

When the bank representative does not recognize your POA: "I have a durable power of attorney on file with this bank. Please verify with your back office. I'll wait." Escalate politely but persistently. Have a copy of the POA on your phone.

When your partner wants to buy something unreasonable: Do not argue about the item. Delay. "Let's sleep on it." The impulse passes. By morning, they will have forgotten. Avoid no. Use not yet.

Reflection Prompts

Which of the seven items in this chapter have you already done? Which have you been putting off, and why?

If you died tomorrow, what is the single most confusing thing your successor would face? Fix that one first.

Who is the attorney, financial planner, or VSO you should be calling next week? When will you call?

What is the most uncomfortable financial conversation you have been avoiding with your partner? What makes it easier to have it sooner rather than later?

The Quick Version

Mental capacity can be lost suddenly in FTD, which means legal and financial work is urgent and must be done while capacity is intact. A durable power of attorney (financial and healthcare), drafted by an elder-law attorney, is the single most important document. All FTD variants are on the Social Security Compassionate Allowances list, which expedites SSDI approval. Medicare does not cover long-term care; Medicaid does, after spend-down. Protecting against disinhibition-driven financial losses requires credit freezes, transaction alerts, separate accounts, and social-media monitoring. Wills, beneficiaries, trusts, and digital asset inventories should be updated now. And you must have a written plan for what happens if you die first.

Chapter 8. Keeping Everyone Safe Together

Paulo got the phone call at 10:17 a.m. on a Wednesday.

It was a woman he did not know, calling from a farm about fifteen miles north of where he and his wife Rita lived. The woman said, carefully, "I have a woman in my kitchen. She says her name is Rita. She says her husband's name is Paulo. She's wearing slippers and a bathrobe. She's been here about forty minutes. She seems confused. I found your number on a little card in her pocket."

Paulo drove to the farm in eleven minutes. He found Rita at the woman's kitchen table drinking tea. Rita looked at him and said, pleasantly, "Oh, hi. Are we going home?"

The card in her pocket was an FTD awareness card Paulo had made six months earlier, after reading about them. It said, "My name is Rita Costa. I have frontotemporal dementia. I may appear confused. Please call my husband Paulo at [number]." Paulo had made five of them. He had put one in each of her jacket pockets, one in her purse, one in her wallet.

Driving home, Paulo realized two things. First, he had almost not made the cards. He had thought it was paranoid. He had thought Rita was not at risk. Second, the cards had just saved her life. She had walked out of the house at 9:30 that morning while Paulo was showering. If the farm's owner had not been kind and observant, Rita could have wandered for hours, or onto a road, or into a pond.

That afternoon he bought a GPS tracker shaped like a watch. He installed door alarms. He printed twenty more cards.

Some partners of people with FTD never have a wandering incident. Some have one. Some have one every three weeks. As FTD progresses, safety issues related to behavior, mobility, and impulse control become a paramount concern, and an environmental and behavioral framework for caregivers tends to be more useful than reliance on the person's own judgment (Talerico & Evans, 2001). This chapter is about building the safety architecture that protects both of you before the incident happens, not after.

Chapter Principle

Safety in FTD is prevention, not supervision. You cannot watch your partner every minute. You can build a system of environmental controls, tracking tools, awareness cards, and pre-planned responses that dramatically reduces the probability of catastrophe. The system is a set of small investments, each of which takes an afternoon to install and may save a life.

8.1 The Driving Conversation No One Wants

Driving is one of the earliest safety risks in FTD, and one of the hardest to address, because driving is tied to identity, independence, and marriage logistics.

The research is clear: most people with FTD should stop driving within the first year or two after diagnosis, and some should stop before diagnosis. Impaired judgment, slowed reaction time, disinhibition, and reduced attention all combine to produce driving risk that is often higher than the person realizes. In some studies, people with FTD have crash rates several times higher than matched controls.

Strategies for the driving conversation:

Get the neurologist to say it. Many states require physicians to report cognitive impairment that affects driving. Some do not, but all neurologists can issue a recommendation. A letter from the neurologist saying "Mr. Costa should no longer drive" lands with authority that yours does not.

Use a formal driving evaluation. Occupational therapists trained in driving rehabilitation can perform on-road evaluations. The evaluation costs several hundred dollars and produces a neutral, third-party recommendation. This takes the decision out of your hands.

Make the car unavailable. Hide the keys. Remove the battery. Sell the car. In some cases, a car that is not visible reduces the demand to drive more than any conversation will.

Offer alternatives. Ride services, family drivers, community transport for older adults. The cessation of driving is a real loss of autonomy. Provide something in its place.

Use AFTD's Driving Agreement. AFTD has a driving contract template that documents the conversation and provides structure. This can help when there is disagreement in the family.

Your partner will be angry about this for a while. Anger is appropriate to the loss. Do not take the car back because of the anger. Drive your partner places yourself if that is what it takes. The risk of someone else's child being killed by your spouse's impaired driving is a risk you cannot recover from.

8.2 Roaming Is Not Wandering

In Alzheimer's, the word is "wandering." The person becomes disoriented, leaves the house, and cannot find their way back. In FTD, the more accurate word is "roaming." People with bvFTD often have preserved navigation skills. They know where they are and how to get home. What they do is walk, or bike, or drive a route, often the same one, repeatedly and compulsively. This is a different phenomenon from wandering, and it requires a different response.

A person roaming is not lost. They are following a compulsion. The destination may be the same coffee shop every day, the same park, the same route along a highway. The risk is not that they cannot find their way home. The risk is that the roaming takes them into traffic, that it happens at times you are not watching, that weather or injury intervenes.

Strategies for roaming:

Know the route. Walk or drive it yourself. Understand the risks. Identify the most dangerous points. Where does the route cross a busy road? Is there a body of water?

Build relationships with people along the route. The coffee shop owner. The gas station attendant. The neighbor on the corner. Give them your number. Tell them about the disease. Ask them to call if your partner seems in trouble.

Accompany when possible. A walking companion may reduce the compulsion or at least make it safer. Family member, friend, hired aide.

Set environmental controls. Door alarms, locked gates, GPS trackers. We cover these in the next section.

Do not try to stop the roaming by force. Compulsions in FTD intensify when blocked. The person may become distressed or aggressive. Work with the compulsion, not against it.

8.3 GPS Trackers, Medical IDs, and FTD Awareness Cards

A handful of inexpensive tools can change the risk profile of a roaming or wandering incident.

GPS trackers. These come in various forms: watches (AngelSense, Theora Care), pendants, shoe inserts, small devices that clip to a belt. Most use cellular data and provide real-time location via an app on your phone. Typical cost is $30 to $300 up front and $10 to $30 monthly. For most families, the value proposition is clear after the first incident.

Medical ID jewelry. A medical alert bracelet or necklace engraved with "Frontotemporal Dementia" and your phone number can be seen by emergency personnel and Good Samaritans. Available from MedicAlert and similar services.

FTD awareness cards. Wallet-sized cards explaining the condition. AFTD offers a free downloadable template. You can also make your own. Include the diagnosis, a request for patience, and your contact information. Keep multiple copies in pockets, purse, car, wallet.

Home location features. If your partner has a smartphone, use Apple's Find My or Google's Find My Device. Keep the phone with them if you can. Charge it.

Registration with local police. Some police departments maintain a voluntary registry of people with cognitive impairment, which can help if they encounter your partner. Check your local department.

8.4 Home Modifications That Prevent Crises

The home is the environment you have the most control over. A handful of modifications dramatically reduce risk.

Door alarms and locks. Simple battery-powered alarms on exterior doors alert you when a door opens. High-mounted deadbolts (above eye level) deter leaving. Do not use them if they would trap your partner in a fire; work with a fire safety consultant if unsure.

Stove safety. Stove knob covers. A gas shutoff valve. Induction cooktops (no flame). Some families disconnect the stove entirely and use a microwave and slow cooker.

Hot water. Set the water heater to 120 degrees Fahrenheit (49 Celsius) or below to prevent scald injuries. Install anti-scald devices on faucets.

Medication lockboxes. All prescription medications, including your partner's, in a lockbox. You are the dispenser. Do not leave pill bottles accessible.

Sharps and tools. Kitchen knives, power tools, yard equipment. Evaluate each based on your partner's specific risks.

Smoke detectors and carbon monoxide detectors. Test them. Replace batteries. Add additional detectors.

Pool and water features. Fence them. Alarm the gates. Water is one of the most common sites of fatal wandering incidents.

Clutter reduction. Falls are a major risk in later FTD. Reduce tripping hazards. Install grab bars in bathrooms. Add night lighting in hallways.

Action Challenge

Walk through your home tonight with a critical eye. Note the top three safety risks you see. Address the most dangerous one within a week. Address the other two within a month. Most home safety modifications cost under $100 and take under an hour to install.

8.5 When Disinhibition Meets Strangers

Public disinhibition can produce uncomfortable moments and, occasionally, legal trouble. Shoplifting, inappropriate touching, traffic violations, aggressive behavior: all have been reported in people with FTD.

Your partner is not a criminal. They have a disease that impairs social judgment. This distinction matters, legally and morally. It also matters in the moment, when you are trying to prevent or de-escalate.

Carry awareness cards. The same cards you use for wandering also defuse disinhibition situations. Hand one to a shop clerk, a server, a police officer. Many people respond with immediate understanding.

Pre-emptively inform venues you visit regularly. The grocery store manager. The server at the regular restaurant. The postal clerk. Sometimes a brief conversation in advance ("my husband has a brain disease that affects his behavior; I wanted to give you a heads up") prevents a future incident from escalating.

Choose settings strategically. Familiar places. Off-peak hours. Shorter outings. Your partner's behavior is usually more predictable when the environment is calm and known.

Leave early. If you see escalation starting, leave. Do not try to finish the meal, the errand, the event. Leaving is not defeat. It is prevention.

8.6 What to Do If Police Get Involved

At some point, police may be called. Someone may call about a wandering incident. A shopkeeper may report shoplifting. A neighbor may call about a disturbance. How you handle the first police contact often shapes everything that follows.

Stay calm and show the FTD card. "My husband has frontotemporal dementia. He is not responsible for his actions in the way you might assume. Here is information about his condition."

Request the officer not interview your partner alone. You are the translator. Your partner cannot reliably explain themselves.

If you are in a jurisdiction with a Crisis Intervention Team (CIT). These are police officers trained in mental health and dementia response. Request a CIT officer if possible.

Document the incident. Officer names, badge numbers, what happened, what was said. You may need this later for insurance, legal, or medical purposes.

Follow up with the neurologist. A legal incident is a clinical event. Report it. It may inform medication changes, supervision levels, or capacity evaluations.

If criminal charges are pursued. Engage an attorney immediately. Many jurisdictions have procedures for diversion when cognitive impairment is documented. The AFTD Helpline can sometimes connect families with attorneys who understand FTD.

From the Person with FTD's Perspective

Your partner, when they wander or behave in ways that raise safety concern, is not being defiant. They are following internal signals that no longer include the safety-check that a healthy brain would perform. They feel, as far as we can tell, that what they are doing is normal or logical in the moment. Afterward, they often do not remember it.

This means the conversation "don't do that again" has little traction. The protective work is upstream of the behavior, in the environment and the tools you build. You are not punishing your partner by putting door alarms on the house. You are adapting the world around a brain that no longer does its own safety work.

Rita, when Paulo brought her home from the farm, did not seem to understand why it was a problem. She said, pleasantly, "I went for a walk." For her, in the moment, that was the whole of the experience. The thirty-degree weather, the bathrobe, the two-hour absence, these were not factored in.

From the Supporting Partner's Perspective

You will feel, sometimes, that you are running a small institution. You have locked doors, GPS trackers, cards in pockets, backup plans, designated contacts at businesses you frequent. You will feel, some mornings, that you cannot possibly keep all these systems running.

You do not need to. You need enough redundancy that one failure does not cascade. The door alarm backs up your attention. The GPS tracker backs up the door alarm. The FTD card backs up the GPS tracker. No single system needs to be perfect. The combination is what keeps both of you safe.

Paulo, in retrospect, said the day of the farm phone call was the worst of his caregiver life, and also, in an odd way, a gift. "It told me exactly where the gaps were. Before that day I had been doing safety as theory. After that day I did it as a system."

Practical Strategies and Scripts

When a family member says you are overreacting to safety concerns: "The AFTD and the neurologist both recommend these measures. You are welcome to stay with him for a weekend and see the day-to-day. I'd appreciate the break."

When your partner resists wearing the GPS watch: "The doctor wants us to track your blood pressure with this." (A harmless reframe. The watch does not need to be named honestly.) Or: "I want to be able to find you if we get separated when we're out together." Tie it to a shared goal.

When police arrive for a wandering incident: "Thank you for calling me. He has frontotemporal dementia. Here's a card explaining. I'm so grateful you found him. Can you help me get him to the car?"

When you forget to lock something and something happens: Forgive yourself fast. You are not a perfect system. You are a human running a difficult system under fatigue. The point is not to avoid all incidents. The point is to reduce their frequency and severity.

Reflection Prompts

What is the safety risk in your household you have been most avoiding addressing? What makes it hard?

Who in your partner's daily environment (neighbors, shopkeepers, regular places) should know about the FTD? Who could you tell this week?

If an incident happened tomorrow, do you have a written plan? If not, could you draft one in an hour this weekend?

What safety intervention would free up your own vigilance the most? That is the one to install first.

The Quick Version

Safety in FTD is about prevention through environmental design, not supervision through attention. Driving should usually stop within the first year or two, and the conversation is easier when the neurologist leads it. Roaming (compulsive, familiar routes) is different from wandering (disorientation) and requires route-specific planning. GPS trackers, medical IDs, and FTD awareness cards are inexpensive tools that change outcomes. Home modifications (door alarms, locked medications, stove controls, water temperature limits) take an afternoon and prevent most common crises. Police interactions are best handled with the awareness card in hand and a calm explanation of the disease. Every safety layer backs up the others; no single layer has to be perfect.

PART THREE: HOLDING ONTO YOURSELF AND THE RELATIONSHIP

Part Three is about the interior of caregiving. It is about what happens to you, to the marriage, to the family, in the slow unfolding of a disease that does not stop. The practical work of Part Two (the lockboxes, the POA, the GPS tracker) keeps both of you safe. The work of Part Three keeps both of you whole.

These five chapters take on the things partners rarely say out loud. The grief that has no funeral. The intimacy that keeps changing shape. The children who know more than you told them. The help you cannot ask for. The body of your own that you have stopped paying attention to.

None of this is optional. Partners who survive the long arc of FTD do not survive it by being saints. They survive it by being honest about what it costs, by building systems of support before they collapse, and by accepting that loving someone with FTD changes who you are, and that change is allowed.

Chapter 9. Grieving Someone Still Here

Adebayo's wife Ngozi had been a high school principal for twenty-two years when she was diagnosed with bvFTD at age fifty-eight. Three years later, she was home full-time, and Adebayo was doing most of the cooking, shopping, and bathing.

One Saturday morning, Adebayo went to a funeral. A colleague from his law firm had died suddenly of a heart attack. The service was at a Catholic church near their home. Adebayo had not been to a funeral in years. He sat in the pew and watched the widow and the two adult children weeping in the front row. Friends and family came up to them afterward. People hugged them. People brought casseroles.

Adebayo drove home and sat in the car in his driveway for forty-five minutes. He finally went inside. Ngozi was on the couch, watching cartoons, eating a bowl of cereal. She did not look up when he came in. She had not noticed he was gone.

That night, after she was asleep, Adebayo sat in his office and wept for the first time in two years. What he finally articulated, to himself, in the dark, was this: *my wife is gone, and there will be no funeral. Nobody is bringing me a casserole. I am the widow of a woman who is asleep upstairs.*

That was the moment he understood what a therapist had been trying to tell him for months. The word she had used was *ambiguous loss*.

Chapter Principle

In FTD, you lose your partner before you lose your partner. The grief starts years before the death. It has no casserole, no service, no closure. It is grief without end markers, and that is what makes it different from any other kind. This chapter is about how to recognize what you are feeling, how to hold it, and how to keep living inside it without being destroyed by it.

9.1 What Pauline Boss Named Decades Ago

Pauline Boss is a family therapist and researcher who spent fifty years studying what she calls ambiguous loss. The concept came from her work with families of soldiers missing in action, where a loved one is physically absent but psychologically present in the family's mind. Later she extended the concept in the other direction, to dementia, where a loved one is physically present but psychologically absent (Boss, 2011).

In her framing, ambiguous loss is the hardest grief humans experience. Ordinary grief has a clear beginning and a slow end. Someone dies. You grieve. Time does its slow work. Ambiguous loss has no clear beginning, no clear end, and no social recognition. The person is here and not here. You cannot close the door. You cannot not close the door. You cannot even fully name what is happening, because the person you are grieving will come downstairs for dinner tonight.

What Boss observed, across hundreds of families, is that ambiguous loss tends to produce a specific set of symptoms that look nothing like stages of grief. It produces what she calls *frozen grief*, the inability to mourn because there is nothing to mourn yet and everything to mourn already. It produces chronic sorrow, which comes in waves rather than a trajectory. It produces a kind of dissociation, where the caregiver's life splits into two tracks: the daily track of making sandwiches and paying bills, and the emotional track that cannot be integrated into ordinary consciousness.

If you have been feeling like your grief has no shape, no progress, no direction, you are not failing at mourning. You are experiencing exactly what Boss documented. The grief is not broken. The situation is unusual, and ordinary grief does not fit it.

9.2 Why FTD Grief Feels Disorganized

FTD grief has features that make it, in many ways, harder than the grief of Alzheimer's caregivers. Studies of FTD-specific caregiver burden have repeatedly shown high rates of depression, anxiety, and social isolation, often higher than those reported among Alzheimer's caregiver groups, with behavioral changes in particular being a key driver of caregiver distress (de Vugt et al., 2006; Diehl-Schmid et al., 2013; Mioshi et al., 2009; Mioshi et al., 2013; Nunnemann et al., 2012; Riedijk et al., 2006).

Three things make FTD grief specifically hard.

First, the personality changes create a particular kind of betrayal-feeling grief. Your partner says cruel things. Your partner stops showing affection. Your partner forgets your birthday. Every one of these events registers, at some level, as abandonment, even when you know intellectually that it is the disease. Your nervous system does not care what you know intellectually. It registers the absence as rejection.

Second, the younger age of onset means you are often losing a partner in midlife, when you were supposed to be planning retirement travel, watching grandchildren grow up, entering the late phase of the marriage together. Instead you are watching a career end early, a future shrink, and social circles thin out. The grief is not just for the person. It is for the entire future you thought you had.

Third, the lack of social recognition amplifies everything. When someone's spouse has cancer or a stroke, friends and family understand. Meals appear. Support shows up. When someone's spouse has FTD, people often do not understand the disease, are uncomfortable visiting, and withdraw. You are grieving a disease most people have never heard of, for a loss that has not happened yet, with almost no social support.

This is why so many FTD caregivers describe feeling invisible. Your grief is invisible to most of your social circle, because the grief has no event to hang on.

9.3 Holding Both The Person Then And Now

One of the hardest tasks of ambiguous loss is holding both versions of your partner in your mind simultaneously: the person you married, and the person you are now caring for. These two people are the same person, and also, in many real ways, not the same person.

Families try to resolve this tension in two directions, both of which tend to cause problems.

One direction is to insist that the person you married is still there, underneath, and the disease is a mask. This is comforting in the short run and often untenable in the long run, because the evidence in front of you contradicts it daily. When your husband laughs at someone's death, it is hard to maintain that the gentle man you married is "still in there."

The other direction is to declare that the person you married is gone and the current person is a stranger. This feels protective, because it reduces the pain of each new loss. It also makes it hard to feed the current person breakfast, which you still have to do.

Both directions are partial truths. The honest position is harder. Your partner is the same person, biologically and historically. They are also, functionally, a different person than the one you married, because specific brain regions that made them who they were have changed. You are caring for someone who is both. You love both. You grieve one while still living with the other.

This dual-consciousness is exhausting to maintain. It is also, in Boss's framing, the only position that actually fits the situation. Everything else is simplification that will eventually collide with reality.

Action Challenge

Write down one specific memory of your partner from before the disease. Make it sensory. What they wore, what they said, what you smelled, where you were. Then write down one thing about your partner today that is still recognizably them. Keep both pages. You will return to them.

9.4 Anticipatory Grief Is Real Grief

You may have heard the term *anticipatory grief*, which describes mourning that begins before the actual death. In FTD, anticipatory grief is not a rehearsal. It is the main event. The death at the end of FTD is often, for the spouse, less acute than the slow losses of the preceding years. Many partners describe the actual death as almost anticlimactic, because they have been losing their person in pieces for so long.

Research on anticipatory grief has, for decades, suggested that it is protective, that grieving before the death reduces the acute grief afterward. More recent research has complicated this picture. Some caregivers do experience less acute grief after the death. Others experience severe grief after the death, on top of the years of anticipatory grief, in a way that cannot be subtracted from one another.

What this means practically is that you cannot "get ahead" of grief by grieving early. You cannot bank anticipatory grief as a credit against the grief to come. The grief you are feeling now is real. The grief that will come when your partner dies will also be real. They will not cancel out.

The corollary is this: do not shame yourself for grieving now. Do not tell yourself "I should save this for when it really happens." This is when it is really happening. You are allowed to grieve a living person who has already been lost in ways that matter.

9.5 Feelings You Are Not Supposed To Have

Caregiver support groups, when they are good, produce a specific kind of relief: the relief of hearing someone else admit to a feeling you have been hiding.

The feelings most commonly hidden:

Relief. When your partner naps, when respite care takes them for a weekend, when an illness means they are quieter than usual. The relief registers as guilt. It is not guilt. It is a normal response to sustained strain.

Anger. Sometimes at your partner, even though you know it is the disease. Sometimes at family members who disappeared. Sometimes at friends who are still living the life you were supposed to be living.

Envy. Of widows who get to grieve cleanly. Of couples still on cruises. Of the neighbors whose biggest problem is their teenager's grades.

Wishing for the end. This is the feeling most hidden and most common. At some point, most long-term FTD caregivers have the thought: *I wish this would end*. Sometimes the thought is about your partner. Sometimes about yourself. Sometimes about both.

None of these feelings makes you a bad person. All of them are common. Researchers who study long-term caregivers find that the thought "I wish this would end" is reported by a majority of spouses caring for someone with advanced dementia. It is a reasonable response to a situation that is not sustainable at its current intensity.

What matters is not that you have these feelings. It is what you do with them. The partners who survive do not suppress them. They do not act on them in harmful ways. They name them to someone they trust, and then they go make dinner.

9.6 Giving Grief A Container Without Closure

Ambiguous loss does not have natural containers. There is no funeral. There is no anniversary of death, because there is no death. There is no closure, which means there is also no official beginning.

Partners who do well often build their own containers, small and imperfect.

A weekly grief hour. Same time, same day. You sit with it for an hour. Cry, write, look at photos, do whatever grief wants. Then the hour ends, and you do something grounding: a walk, a meal, a call to a friend.

A document of losses. Some partners keep a running log of specific things lost. "December 3: the last time he called me 'honey.'" "February 14: she did not remember it was our anniversary." The document becomes a record of the grief that has no public marker. It is not morbid. It is witnessing.

Rituals for the milestones that have no marker. The day you moved from the bedroom because their sleep was too disturbed. The day you took over the finances. The day the neurologist said "moderate." Light a candle. Say a prayer. Write a letter you do not send. Mark the thing that had no one else to mark it.

A therapist or support group attuned to ambiguous loss. Most therapists are trained in ordinary grief. Fewer are trained in ambiguous loss. When you find one who gets it, hold on.

The point is not to reach closure. Closure is not available to you. The point is to let the grief have somewhere to go, so it does not leak into every ordinary moment.

From the Person with FTD's Perspective

People with FTD, especially bvFTD, often experience reduced emotional depth as a feature of the disease. Loss of sympathy or empathy and emotional blunting are core diagnostic features of bvFTD (Rascovsky et al., 2011). This means your partner may not experience their own losses the way you would expect.

This is heartbreaking in one direction and merciful in another. Your partner may not be grieving the disease the way you are. They may not be tracking what they have lost. They may not miss their own old self. In Boss's framing, this is part of what makes the loss ambiguous. The person is losing things they cannot mourn, so you are left to mourn for both of you.

For people with PPA, who often retain insight, grief is more present. Many PPA patients describe sadness, frustration, and anticipatory grief of their own. If your partner has preserved awareness, they may be carrying their own grief alongside yours. It is worth asking gently, when the moment is right.

From the Supporting Partner's Perspective

The grief will not be linear. It will come in waves that do not correspond to anything external. You will cry in a hardware store. You will be fine at the funeral of your own father. You will have a peaceful week followed by a devastating Tuesday for no reason you can identify.

This is not you falling apart. This is how ambiguous loss moves. The research on grief, updated since Kübler-Ross, no longer supports the idea of clean stages that complete in order. Grief is recursive. It circles back to where you have already been. It surprises you. It does not finish.

Adebayo, three years after his funeral-epiphany, said this in a support group: "I stopped expecting to be done. I just stopped. Once I stopped expecting to be done, the grief got easier to carry. It was the expectation of completion that was making it worse."

Practical Strategies and Scripts

When someone says "but she's still here, you should be grateful": "I am grateful. And I'm also grieving. Both things are true. I need you to let both things be true."

When you feel relief that your partner is napping and the relief feels wrong: Name it out loud, to yourself or to one trusted person. "I'm relieved he's napping. That's allowed. Relief is not betrayal. It's oxygen."

When you cannot stop crying: Set a timer. Fifteen minutes. Let yourself cry fully. When the timer rings, drink a full glass of water, stand up, and do one concrete task. The container does not stop the grief. It keeps the grief from colonizing the whole day.

When a friend disappears because they cannot handle the disease: Do not chase. Do not explain. Grieve the friendship quietly and move your limited energy toward the people who stayed.

Reflection Prompts

What loss has happened in the last year that nobody but you noticed?

Which of the "forbidden" feelings (relief, anger, envy, wishing for the end) have you had? What would it mean to let yourself have it without judgment?

What is one container you could build this month to hold your grief on purpose?

Who is one person you could tell, honestly, how you are actually doing?

The Quick Version

Ambiguous loss, named by Pauline Boss, is grief for someone physically present but psychologically absent. It has no funeral, no social recognition, and no natural container. FTD grief is particularly hard because of personality changes, early age of onset, and low public awareness. Holding both the person your partner was and the person they are now is exhausting, and also the only honest position. Anticipatory grief is real grief, not a rehearsal, and it does not cancel the grief that comes after the death. The "forbidden" feelings (relief, anger, envy, wishing for the end) are common and do not make you a bad partner. Grief without closure needs containers you build yourself, because the world will not provide them.

Chapter 10. Love When Everything Shifts

Marco had not touched his wife Ana in seven months.

Not in the way they used to touch each other. He still helped her bathe. He still buttoned her cardigan in the mornings. He still kissed her forehead when she fell asleep on the couch in the afternoons. But the bed, which had been for thirty-one years a place of warmth and reach and easy physical conversation, had become a place where two people slept with their backs to each other.

It was not Ana's fault. Her bvFTD had flattened her affection. She did not initiate anymore. She did not respond when he initiated. The absence was not hostile. It was absent the way a room is absent of someone who has moved out. Marco had tried, twice, to talk to her about it. She had looked at him politely and said, "I don't know what you mean, Marco," and then asked what was for dinner.

One Tuesday night, late, Marco was half-asleep. Ana, asleep beside him, rolled over and without waking, found his hand under the blanket and took it. She held it for perhaps ten seconds. Then she rolled back over.

Marco lay awake for the rest of the night. What broke something in him was not the holding. It was that she had done it in her sleep. Whatever was still there, whatever had reached for him, had come from below the disease. It was still there. He had been assuming it was gone, and it was not gone. The machinery for expressing it was broken. The thing itself was not.

In the morning, he made coffee. He sat across from Ana at the kitchen table. She ate her cereal. She did not look at him in the way she used to. But when he reached across the table and put his hand over hers, she did not pull away. She looked down at the hands, together, and smiled a small smile that might have meant nothing, and might have meant something. Marco decided, that morning, that the difference did not matter as much as he had thought.

Chapter Principle

Intimacy does not end when the disease changes the way it used to look. The channels for expression narrow, and the forms shift, but something underneath usually persists. The work is to find what is still there, to protect the forms that still function, and to stop measuring the current relationship against the one you used to have.

10.1 Redefining Intimacy When Words Go

Intimacy is not one thing. It is a collection of practices, many of which happen without conscious attention: the way you finish each other's sentences, the inside jokes, the specific way your partner says your name, the brief touches as you pass in the kitchen, the sexual life, the way you debrief about the day in bed at night. In FTD, some of these channels break down. Others change shape. A few, sometimes, persist almost unchanged.

The partners who adapt well to the changing terrain of intimacy tend to do two things. They mourn the channels that are gone without pretending they are not gone. And they invest actively in the channels that still work.

If your partner with PPA can no longer banter, you do not have banter anymore. Mourn the banter. Then notice what else is still available. Maybe they still hold your hand while watching TV. Maybe they still smile when you come home from the grocery store. Maybe they still laugh at specific old videos of the grandchildren. Whatever is still there, name it, and spend more time in it.

If your partner with bvFTD has become affectively flat, the old forms of emotional reciprocity may be gone. But physical presence, shared meals, shared music, shared rituals may still register.

Research on attachment in advanced dementia suggests that even people who show no overt response to family members often have elevated physiological markers of recognition when a spouse enters the room. Something underneath the flatness is still tracking you.

10.2 Sex, Hypersexuality, and Honest Conversations

Sexual changes in FTD are common, real, and almost never discussed openly. They fall into two broad patterns, and your partner may show either or both.

Hypersexuality is increased sexual drive, reduced inhibition around sexual behavior, or inappropriate sexual behavior in public. It is more common in bvFTD, particularly when the right orbitofrontal cortex is affected. It can include inappropriate comments, touching of strangers, excessive pornography use, or sexual demands on the partner that do not match the previous relationship dynamic. It is a symptom of the disease, not a revelation of hidden desire. It is also, in some cases, a safety and legal issue that requires intervention.

Hyposexuality and reduced affection is the opposite pattern, where sexual interest, responsiveness, and affection decline or disappear. This is more common in the later stages of bvFTD and across PPA. It is the pattern Marco was experiencing with Ana. It is often devastating to the partner, because the absence of physical affection reads emotionally as rejection, even when you know it is the disease.

Both patterns raise hard questions about consent, dignity, and the partner's own sexual needs over a long arc. There are no easy answers. A few principles help.

Sexual consent requires capacity. As your partner's cognitive function declines, there will come a point where they can no longer meaningfully consent to sexual activity. Where exactly that point sits is individual and ethically complex. Many long-term couples work with a neurologist or specialist in dementia-informed sexuality to think this through. The Alzheimer's Society in the UK has a good primer on consent and intimacy in dementia that applies well to FTD.

Your needs as the caregiver-partner are real. Many long-term FTD caregivers describe sexual loneliness as one of the least-spoken hardships of the disease. Some couples, with open communication established earlier, agree on an arrangement where the well partner has other outlets. Others find that the sexual life ends and they grieve it. There is no right answer. There are only honest conversations with yourself and, if you are fortunate, with a therapist who understands both dementia and sexuality.

Disinhibited sexual behavior in public may require environmental management (the same principles as Chapter 5) and medication. If your partner is touching strangers, masturbating in public, or making sexual comments that put them at legal risk, talk to the neurologist. SSRIs and, in some cases, hormonal treatments can reduce these behaviors.

10.3 Touch Music Food And The Senses That Remain

When verbal intimacy becomes difficult, non-verbal channels take on disproportionate weight. This is not a consolation prize. The non-verbal channels were always there. You are just being asked to rely on them more consciously.

Touch. Hand-holding, back rubs, hair stroking, a hand on the shoulder while walking past. Research on touch in dementia care consistently shows that gentle, predictable, consensual touch reduces agitation, lowers cortisol, and increases oxytocin release in both the person receiving and the person giving. It is, in a measurable sense, a physiological intimacy. It works even when the person can no longer respond in words.

Music. The research on music and dementia is extensive and remarkable. Familiar music from the person's young adulthood frequently produces recognizable responses, even in late disease. Playlists built from songs your partner loved in their twenties and thirties, played at consistent times, become both intimacy and medicine. Moments of recognition, of a foot tapping, of a mouthed lyric, are not trivial. They are the person, still accessible, under the disease.

Food. Shared meals are one of the oldest human forms of intimacy. In FTD, eating preferences often change (Chapter 5), but the ritual of eating together can often be preserved. Same table, same time, same basic shape of a meal. Your partner's body remembers this, even when their mind has let go of the details.

Smell. Familiar smells (the soap your partner always used, a specific perfume, the shampoo of a loved one) often retain emotional weight longer than verbal memory. Smell has a direct neural path to the limbic system that bypasses much of the damage of FTD.

Action Challenge

This week, identify one non-verbal channel of intimacy that is still available (touch, music, food, routine) and intentionally deepen it. Play the Saturday morning album every Saturday morning. Hold hands during every evening TV show. Eat breakfast at the same table, every day, without phones. The point is not to perform intimacy. It is to protect the channels that still work from being lost to neglect.

10.4 What Marriage Means When Consent Blurs

At some point in many FTD arcs, the partner without the disease becomes, functionally, the decision-maker for both. This shift is gradual. It is not a single moment. It happens in increments: the first decision you make for your partner about their clothes, about their appointments, about their money, about their medical care, about where they live, about if they will have surgery.

The marriage changes in this shift. You are still married. You are also, functionally, a fiduciary of the other person's life. Most marriage vows do not anticipate this. They still cover it.

What changes in practice:

You speak for your partner in medical appointments. Their voice, when present, is one input; you are the interpreter.

You make decisions your partner would have had a say in. You will often not know what they would have wanted. You make your best guess based on decades of knowing them.

You become responsible for your partner's dignity in ways they can no longer advocate for themselves: how they are dressed, how they are spoken to, how they are treated by medical staff, if strangers understand they were once someone else.

You become the guardian of their story. You are the person who remembers, on their behalf, what they used to believe, what they used to want, who they used to be.

This expanded role is exhausting and sometimes isolating. It is also, in the long arc of love, a kind of late fidelity. Standing in for someone who can no longer stand in for themselves is one of the oldest things marriages do.

10.5 Finding Small Moments That Still Feel Like You

Most long-term FTD caregivers, when asked what keeps them in the relationship, describe small specific moments rather than grand ones. They describe moments where the relationship felt, briefly, recognizable.

Marco, months after his middle-of-the-night revelation, kept a running list on his phone of moments he called "glimpses." The list included:

Tuesday, 7:15 a.m. Ana laughed at a squirrel outside the kitchen window the way she used to laugh at squirrels.

Saturday, 3:00 p.m. Ana sang along to the chorus of a Fleetwood Mac song on the radio, the first time she had sung in five months.

Wednesday, 9:30 p.m. When I kissed her goodnight, she kissed me back, briefly, before she turned over.

The glimpses were rare, scattered, and unpredictable. They were also, for Marco, evidence that something he had been grieving as entirely lost was not entirely lost. They did not change the arc of the disease. They did not even happen often enough to provide reliable comfort. But they happened, and he wrote them down, and on the hardest days he read the list, and it helped.

You will have your own glimpses. They will be specific to your relationship. They will not come on demand, and you cannot force them. What you can do is notice them when they happen, write them down, and let them be evidence.

10.6 Loneliness Inside The Relationship

One of the hardest things about long-term FTD caregiving is the specific loneliness of being married to someone who is no longer the person you married. You can be lonely in an empty house. You can be lonelier in a house with someone who does not turn to you the way they used to.

Name this loneliness. It is not a failure of love. It is a feature of the situation. Long-term partners of people with advanced dementia describe loneliness rates that approach those of recently bereaved widows and widowers.

The responses that help, in no particular order: friendships that existed before the disease, if any have been maintained. A regular therapist or support group. A spiritual community, if that is your orientation. Creative work that belongs only to you. Physical affection from people who understand the limits (adult children, close friends, a pet). Writing. Walks alone.

What does not help: pretending the loneliness is not there. Shaming yourself for feeling it. Expecting your partner to fill it. They cannot.

From the Person with FTD's Perspective

What does your partner experience in the intimate space of the marriage? The honest answer is that we do not fully know, and it varies enormously by variant and stage.

In bvFTD, emotional flatness is often accompanied by reduced awareness of the partner's emotional state. Your partner may not notice that you are distant, sad, or hurt. This is not cruelty. The circuits that would have noticed are damaged. If your partner is not responding to your emotional cues, they are not ignoring them. They are not receiving them.

In PPA, where emotional awareness is often preserved, your partner may be acutely aware of the changes in the relationship and may be grieving them in parallel with you. They may also be unable to articulate this grief, which can read from the outside as absence.

In either case, your partner's brain is not running a hidden inner life of rejection of you. They are not withholding intimacy. They are, in different ways, struggling to generate or express it. What remains, underneath, may be much more intact than the surface suggests.

From the Supporting Partner's Perspective

You are allowed to have needs that your partner can no longer meet. You are allowed to grieve the sexual life of the marriage. You are allowed to miss being flirted with. You are allowed to want to be seen, desired, challenged, and met.

These wants do not make you disloyal. They make you a living human being whose partner has a disease that affects the parts of them that used to meet those wants. The disease is not a referendum on your worth or attractiveness. It is a disease.

Marco, five years into Ana's bvFTD, said this to a newer caregiver: "I stopped waiting for her to be my partner in the way she used to be. I started being her partner in the way she needs now. Somewhere in that shift, I stopped being as lonely. Not fully. Just less."

Practical Strategies and Scripts

When your partner stops initiating affection: Do not wait for them to initiate. Initiate yourself, small and predictable. Hand on shoulder, kiss on forehead, back rub at bedtime. Build rituals that do not require their initiation.

When you feel sexually lonely: Talk to a therapist trained in dementia and sexuality. This is more common than people assume and less shameful than you fear. Therapists can help you work through the ethics and the practicalities without judgment.

When your partner exhibits disinhibited sexual behavior in public: Remove your partner from the setting. Apologize briefly to anyone affected. Do not punish or lecture your partner. Discuss with the neurologist about behavioral and medication approaches.

When a friend asks "is the marriage still a marriage?": "It is different. The shape has changed. It is still the marriage. I am still his wife. He is still my husband. The content has shifted, not the container."

Reflection Prompts

What non-verbal channel of intimacy is still working in your relationship? How often are you using it intentionally?

What have you been grieving as "gone" that might still be accessible if you invested in it differently?

What is your own need for touch, affection, and being seen, and who in your life can meet that need in appropriate ways?

When was the last glimpse? What happened? What did you notice?

The Quick Version

Intimacy in FTD does not end, but the channels for it narrow and shift. Mourn the channels that are gone, and invest actively in the ones that still work. Sexual changes in FTD fall into two patterns (hypersexuality and hyposexuality), both of which are symptoms rather than expressions of the person. Touch, music, food, smell, and routine persist as channels of connection far into the disease. Marriage vows were not written for this, but they still cover it; you become, functionally, the fiduciary of both lives. Glimpses of the person your partner used to be still happen; write them down. Loneliness inside the relationship is real, does not mean you have stopped loving your partner, and deserves its own support.

Chapter 11. Telling Children What Is Happening

Maya was eleven when her father was diagnosed with bvFTD. Her mother Priya did not tell her for six months. Priya told herself she was waiting until she knew more, until she could explain it properly, until Maya seemed ready. What Priya did not realize was that Maya already knew something was wrong. Maya had known for longer than Priya had.

Maya had noticed her father no longer laughed at her jokes. She had noticed he had stopped helping her with math. She had noticed he sometimes said mean things to her mother at dinner and then looked confused when her mother cried. She had noticed her mother crying in the laundry room. She had noticed her own friends had stopped being invited over, because she could not predict what her father would say.

One Sunday afternoon, when Priya was in the kitchen, Maya came in and sat at the table. She said, "Mom. What is wrong with Dad?"

Priya froze. She had imagined this conversation for six months. She had rehearsed it. She had planned to use words like "the doctors are still figuring it out." She had planned to buy time.

Instead, she sat down across from Maya and said, "His brain is sick. There's a disease that's changing how he acts. It's called frontotemporal dementia. It's not going away. I should have told you sooner, and I'm sorry."

Maya cried. Then Maya said, "Okay. Thank you for telling me."

That night Priya called the child psychologist who had been recommended by her neurologist's social worker. The psychologist said what many pediatric psychologists say in these situations:

children always know, because they watch, and they are attuned to their parents. The question is not if you should tell them. It is if they have permission to talk about what they already know.

Chapter Principle

Children notice long before you tell them. Secrecy does not protect them; it isolates them. Age-appropriate honesty, delivered calmly and continuously, is the single best predictor of how children do in a family with parental illness. This chapter is about what to say, at what age, and how to keep the conversation open as the disease progresses.

11.1 What Kids Pick Up That You Think You Hid

Pediatric psychology has been consistent on this point for decades: children in families with a seriously ill parent pick up more than adults assume. They notice changes in tone, in routine, in who is crying, in which topics are forbidden at dinner. They notice the whispered phone calls. They notice the appointments their parents try to hide.

What children do with this information depends on having a framework. Without a framework, children tend to construct their own explanations, and the explanations children construct are often worse than the truth. Common self-generated explanations include: the parents are getting divorced, the ill parent hates me, I did something to cause this, I am about to be abandoned.

A framework, even a simple one, displaces these fears. "Dad has a brain disease. It makes him act differently. It is not your fault. It is not my fault. It is not going to go away. We are going to love each other through it." This framework does not eliminate the fear. It contains it.

Qualitative research on children and young people who have a parent with young-onset dementia describes the strain of secrecy, the burden of caring without language for what is happening, and the value of being included in honest, age-appropriate conversations (Allen et al., 2009; Svanberg et al., 2010). Children who are told early and allowed to ask questions over time tend to feel less isolated than children whose parents tried to protect them by hiding the illness; the protection often backfires, because the child is left to work out what is happening alone.

11.2 Scripts By Age From Five To Fifteen

The language you use depends on the child's age and developmental stage. The underlying message stays the same. Here are starting points.

Ages 4 to 7. Concrete, simple, present-focused. "Daddy's brain is sick. It makes him act different sometimes. It's not because he doesn't love you. It's because of the sick part of his brain. Doctors are helping him. Mommy is going to take care of him and you. If you have questions, you can always ask me."

Children this age do not need the word *frontotemporal*. They need the word *sick*, the word *brain*, and the promise that someone is taking care of things. Repeat the conversation as needed. They will forget. That is okay. They will ask again.

Ages 8 to 12. More detail, more room for questions, more acknowledgment of how this affects them. "Dad has a disease called frontotemporal dementia. It's a disease that changes his brain over time. It's making him act differently and forget words. Doctors cannot cure it. I'm going to tell you what's happening as it changes, because you deserve to know. You can ask me anything. Some of this is going to be hard. We'll handle it together."

Children this age may want to research it. Let them. The AFTD website has age-appropriate materials. Limit doomscrolling by pre-selecting good resources.

Ages 13 to 18. Full information, full agency, and honesty about uncertainty. "This is what the disease is. This is what we know. This is what we don't know. This is what it means for our family. This is what we expect to change in the next year. I need to know what you need. I need to know when you're struggling. You can have your own feelings about this that are different from mine, and that's okay. We're on the same team."

Teens often need permission to have their own grief, their own anger, their own embarrassment. They also need some protection from being conscripted into caregiving. More on this in 11.5.

11.3 Teens Shame and The Friend Group Problem

Teenagers have a specific pain in an FTD household, and it is worth naming directly: the pain of a parent whose behavior is unpredictable in public, and the impossibility of explaining this to fourteen-year-old friends.

Your teenager may stop inviting friends over. They may stop bringing dates home. They may avoid being seen in public with the parent who has FTD. This is not disloyalty. It is adolescent development colliding with a disease that makes their parent embarrassing in ways your teenager cannot control.

Strategies that help:

Acknowledge the shame without shaming them for it. "I know it's hard to bring friends home. You don't have to apologize for that. It's a real thing." This is different from "you shouldn't feel embarrassed." The first validates. The second denies.

Offer alternatives. Meet friends outside the house. Hold social events at times when the ill parent is sleeping or at adult day care. Let your teenager have a zone of their life that is not defined by the disease.

Give them language. If they want to tell a friend, help them script it. "My dad has a kind of dementia. It makes him act weird sometimes. I don't want to talk about it a lot. I just wanted you to know." Friends who matter will understand. Friends who do not understand, at fourteen, may not be the ones worth investing in anyway.

Protect their social life. Do not use your teenager as primary caregiving support when there are other options. Their adolescence is happening once. Do not borrow it.

11.4 Adult Children and Blended Family Reality

Adult children bring different challenges than younger kids. They are often geographically distant. They may have their own families and careers. They may have complicated feelings about the parent who is ill, especially if the parent was difficult before the disease.

Blended families add a layer. If your partner has children from a prior marriage, those children may have their own relationship with the parent and their own caregiving role, sometimes in tension with yours. The Willis family, with Emma Heming Willis and Bruce Willis's adult daughters from his first marriage with Demi Moore, is a visible example of how this can work well when there is goodwill on all sides.

Principles for adult children and blended families:

Communicate directly and regularly. Not through other people. If your stepdaughter needs to know something, you tell her, or your partner tells her when they can. Do not route information through intermediaries.

Share the work if they want to share it. Some adult children want to help. Let them. Assign specific tasks. Vague offers of help tend to dissipate. Specific requests get done.

Do not demand help from those who cannot give it. Some adult children live across the country. Some have young children of their own. Some have strained relationships with the ill parent. You cannot extract caregiving from resentment. Let them do what they can.

Make room for their grief. Adult children are losing a parent. Their grief is real, even if it looks different from yours. Do not dismiss it. Do not compete with it.

Handle the inheritance questions carefully. Blended families often have legacy and inheritance complexities that get worse under the stress of illness. An estate attorney familiar with blended families is worth the money.

11.5 When Children Become Caregivers Too

In many FTD families, children end up doing caregiving work. Sometimes this is unavoidable. Sometimes it is harmful to the child. Knowing the difference is part of your job as the well parent.

Appropriate child participation includes: being kind to the ill parent, helping with small age-appropriate tasks, understanding why changes are happening, being part of family conversations about the disease.

Inappropriate child caregiving includes: being the primary supervisor of the ill parent for long periods, being responsible for managing crises, taking on emotional caregiving of the well parent, sacrificing school or social development to caregiving.

The line between these is not always clear. Economic necessity sometimes pushes families across it. When this happens, seek support. Young caregivers, as the field calls them, have specific resources available in many countries. The AFTD Teens and Young Adults group is a good starting point in the United States.

Signs your child may be taking on too much: grades slipping, friendships withdrawn, sleep changes, anxiety about leaving the house, mood shifts, sudden interest or anxiety about adult topics (finances, medical decisions).

Do not use a child as your emotional primary support. This is a specific mistake grieving spouses make, often without meaning to. A twelve-year-old is not equipped to be your confidant. Find adults for that.

Action Challenge

This week, have one conversation with each child in your household that includes an open-ended question about how they are doing, not just what they need. "How have you been feeling about things with Dad lately?" Then listen without fixing.

11.6 The Genetic Question Kids Eventually Ask

At some point, often in adolescence or early adulthood, the child asks: am I going to get this?

The answer depends on your partner's specific FTD variant, which tests have been done, and if there is a known genetic cause. About 30 to 40 percent of FTD cases have a known genetic component. For children of a parent with a known pathogenic variant in *C9orf72*, *MAPT*, or *GRN*, the inheritance is typically autosomal dominant, meaning each child has a 50 percent chance of inheriting the variant.

Do not lie about this. Do not terrify, either. The conversation should happen with a genetic counselor involved whenever possible.

General principles:

If there is no known genetic cause in your partner's case, the risk to your children is elevated but much smaller than 50 percent. Counselors can give specific numbers based on family history.

If there is a known pathogenic variant, adult children can choose predictive testing, which tells them if they have inherited the variant. This decision is deeply personal and should not be rushed. Many adults choose not to test, especially if there is no treatment to change outcomes. This is a reasonable choice.

Children under 18 generally should not have predictive genetic testing for adult-onset conditions. Most professional guidelines reserve this for adulthood, when the person can make an informed decision.

Insurance and employment implications vary by country. In the United States, the Genetic Information Nondiscrimination Act (GINA) offers some protection but does not cover all insurance types (long-term care, life, disability). Genetic counselors walk families through this.

What children often need, when they ask the question, is less information than you think. They need to know that the question has an answer. They need to know they have the option to find out when they are ready. They need to know that whatever the answer, they are not alone with it.

From the Person with FTD's Perspective

Your partner, in the early stages of the disease, may have strong opinions about what to tell the children. Honor those opinions if they can be safely honored. Their voice in their own illness matters.

As the disease progresses, your partner may lose insight into the effect of their behavior on the children. They may say cruel things to a teenager and not register that the teenager is hurt. They may not understand why a child has stopped visiting. This is not a failure of love. It is the disease.

What tends to persist, in many FTD patients, is physical affection toward children. Your partner may not remember the child's name, but may still brighten when the child enters the room. Keep the children around when it is safe. The physical presence of children often reaches the person when nothing else does.

From the Supporting Partner's Perspective

Telling the children is one of the hardest parts of the early disease, and you are likely going to do some version of it badly, and that is okay. Priya waited six months. Many parents do. The goal is not to do it perfectly. The goal is to open the door and keep it open.

You will have your own grief about your children's childhood being shaped by this disease. Your teenager should not be having these conversations. Your nine-year-old should not be watching this. You did not choose this for them. You cannot prevent it. You can be the one steady presence in their world while everything else shifts.

Priya, two years after her Sunday kitchen conversation with Maya, said: "I thought I was protecting her by not telling her. I was not protecting her. I was protecting me, from having to say it out loud. Once I said it, she was more okay than I was. Children are more resilient than we give them credit for, if we give them the truth and let them come to us."

Practical Strategies and Scripts

When you finally tell a child and they ask a question you cannot answer: "That is a great question. I don't know the answer. I'll find out, and I'll tell you what I learn." Then actually do it.

When a child acts out because of the family stress: Do not assume it is the disease causing the acting out. Sometimes it is. Sometimes it is being eleven. Treat the behavior on its own terms while remembering the context.

When a relative criticizes you for telling the children too much: "The pediatric psychologist and the neurologist both recommended age-appropriate honesty. The research supports it. I appreciate your concern. I have this."

When a child becomes a caregiver in ways you do not want: Have the conversation directly. "I have noticed you are doing a lot for Dad. I am grateful. I am also worried you are taking on too much. Your job right now is to be [age]. Let me carry more of this."

Reflection Prompts

What do you think your children already know that you have not discussed with them?

What is one conversation you have been putting off? What makes it feel impossible? What would make it more possible?

Are any of your children taking on more than is age-appropriate? What could shift to relieve them?

What does your child need that you have not asked about recently?

The Quick Version

Children in FTD families know something is wrong long before they are told. Secrecy creates isolation and worse self-generated explanations. Age-appropriate honesty, delivered calmly and repeatedly, produces the best outcomes. Scripts by age range from simple ("Daddy's brain is sick") for young children to full information and agency for teens. Teenagers face specific social pain and need language, alternatives, and protection from premature caregiving. Adult children and blended families require direct communication, shared work where possible, and careful attention to inheritance and legacy. Children can appropriately participate in caregiving within limits; young caregivers who take on too much show measurable developmental costs. The genetic question will eventually be asked; it should be answered honestly, with a genetic counselor involved, and without rushing children toward testing they are not ready for.

Chapter 12. Building Your Support Team

Frances had been caring for her husband Gerald alone for nineteen months when she passed out in the produce aisle at the grocery store.

The store manager called an ambulance. Frances spent the night in the hospital for dehydration, low blood pressure, and what the ER doctor called "caregiver collapse." Her daughter Sonia drove up from three hours away and stayed for a week. During that week, Sonia learned for the first time how much her mother had been doing. Sonia had assumed, based on Frances's reassurances, that everything was fine.

On the fifth day, Sonia sat her mother down at the kitchen table and said, "Mom. You are going to die doing this. You cannot keep doing this alone. I am going to help you build a team. We are going to start this afternoon."

Frances, who had been saying "I'm fine" to every offer of help for nineteen months, did not argue. She was too tired to argue. She sat at the table and watched her daughter open a spreadsheet.

By the end of the week they had: a cleaning service that came every two weeks. A meal delivery service that brought pre-made dinners three times a week. A home health aide who came for four hours on Tuesdays and Thursdays so Frances could leave the house. Gerald's cousin, who had offered help a year ago and been refused, now took Gerald to lunch every Saturday. Two friends from Frances's church had agreed to take shifts on Sundays. A teenager down the street had been hired to mow the lawn. A social worker at the AFTD-affiliated clinic two towns over had been contacted and was setting up a weekly support group call.

Frances looked at the list. She said to Sonia, "I could have done all of this a year ago."

Sonia said, "Yes. You could have. You did not."

Frances cried. Then she laughed. Then she cried more. She said, "Why didn't I?"

Sonia said, "Because you thought asking for help would make you a failure. It doesn't. It makes you a survivor."

Chapter Principle

You cannot do this alone. Partners who try to carry FTD alone do not last the full arc. They collapse, like Frances, or they quietly burn out and become bitter. Building a support team is not a failure of devotion. It is the infrastructure that makes devotion sustainable. This chapter is about exactly how to build one.

12.1 Why You Keep Saying You Are Fine

Most long-term FTD caregivers spend months or years saying "I'm fine" to every offer of help. The reasons are specific and worth examining, because they are often the first obstacle to building a team.

"It feels like admitting failure." If you accept help, you are acknowledging you cannot do this alone. Accepting that is often the hardest psychological move. Partners who grew up believing that love equals self-sacrifice have to unlearn this framework before they can accept help. Love and help are not opposites. They are partners.

"I don't want to be a burden." This is, in some version, what everyone says. The people who love you want to help you. Denying them the chance to help you is not kindness to them. It is an assumption on your part that they will resent helping, which most of them will not.

"I don't know what to ask for." Many offers of help are vague ("let me know if I can do anything"), and vague offers rarely get taken up, because the person being helped cannot translate them into specifics in a crisis. The solution is not to refuse offers. The solution is to get specific about what you need, which the next section addresses.

"The help won't do it right." Paid or volunteer help may not fold the laundry the way you fold it. They may not make the coffee the way you make it. They may not do it as well as you do. This is often true, and it is still better than you doing everything. Lower your standards for tasks that do not require your specific skills.

"My partner resists strangers in the house." This is a real issue in FTD. Introduce helpers gradually. Have them come when your partner is comfortable. Use them for times when you leave the house rather than as direct care for your partner when possible.

"We can't afford it." Sometimes true. Often less true than it feels. We address the money in 12.6.

12.2 The Specific Ask List

Emma Heming Willis credits a simple technique with transforming her caregiver support: she made a list of specific two-hour tasks that someone could do to help her, and kept the list on her phone. When someone said "let me know if I can help," she had an answer.

The technique works because it does three things. It bypasses the vagueness problem. It lets helpers feel useful in a discrete way. And it takes the cognitive load of "what do I need?" off you in moments of crisis.

Your list might include items like:

Sit with my partner for two hours Saturday afternoon so I can go to a movie.

Pick up groceries from [store] using this list.

Drive my partner to the dentist Tuesday at 10 a.m.

Bring us dinner on Friday.

Fold the laundry that is in the dryer.

Mow the lawn.

Pay the cable bill on the counter.

Walk the dog tonight.

Sit with my partner for three hours Sunday morning so I can go to church.

Come over and do any one task from the kitchen whiteboard without asking.

The key is specificity. "Help out around the house" is not an item. "Mow the lawn" is an item. "Support me emotionally" is not an item. "Take me to lunch Tuesday" is an item.

When someone offers help, read them three items from the list. Let them pick. Do not apologize for the specificity. Specificity is a gift to both of you.

12.3 Finding An FTD-Literate Care Team

Many medical and home care providers have never heard of FTD. Your work is to build a team that either knows the disease or is willing to learn it.

Your neurologist. Should be a behavioral or cognitive neurologist. If the one you have is not specifically trained in FTD, consider if a periodic consultation at a specialty center (UCSF, UPenn, Mayo, Johns Hopkins, Mass General in the US; UCL and Cambridge in the UK) can supplement local care.

Primary care physician. Yours and your partner's. Ideally one who respects the neurologist's recommendations and does not try to override them. Primary care is where routine medical problems get caught, and you cannot afford a PCP who does not understand that your partner is cognitively impaired.

Speech-language pathologist. If your partner has PPA, a speech-language pathologist is essential. They can do communication partner training, assess for AAC, and track progression.

Neuropsychologist. For assessments over time, for capacity evaluations, and for input on behavioral strategies.

Social worker. Often affiliated with memory clinics or hospital systems. Can connect you to community resources, sort through insurance questions, and sometimes provide counseling.

Occupational therapist. Can assess home safety, recommend modifications, and sometimes work on daily living skills.

Geriatric care manager. A licensed professional (usually a nurse or social worker) who coordinates care, advocates in medical settings, and provides crisis response. Expensive but often worth it in complex cases.

Elder law attorney. For POA, wills, trusts, Medicaid planning. Re-reference Chapter 7.

Financial planner familiar with disability. Different from an estate attorney. Helps you build a sustainable financial plan across the arc.

Home health aide or personal care attendant. For direct care. Vet carefully. Introduce gradually. Dementia-specific training is a plus.

Therapist for you. Ideally someone trained in ambiguous loss and caregiver grief. Chapter 13 expands on this.

Not every family needs all of these. Most need more than they think. Start with what you can afford and add as the disease progresses.

12.4 Respite Care Without The Guilt

Respite care means someone else takes over caregiving for a defined period so you can rest. It is not optional. It is a clinical necessity for long-term caregivers.

Respite comes in several forms.

In-home respite. A paid aide or volunteer comes to your home and stays with your partner for hours or a day. Often the least disruptive to your partner, and the easiest for you to arrange.

Adult day programs. Your partner goes to a structured program for a day or part of a day, several times a week. Many programs have dementia-specific tracks. Costs vary; some are subsidized.

Short-term residential respite. Your partner goes to a memory care facility for a few days or a week. This allows you to actually leave town. Many facilities offer this.

Family respite. A relative takes your partner for a weekend. Depends on family capacity and your partner's comfort with the relative.

The guilt around respite is universal and specific. Common thoughts: "I should be able to do this myself." "My partner will be distressed without me." "I don't deserve a break."

None of these is accurate. You cannot do this alone. Your partner will adapt. You absolutely deserve a break, and more than that, your partner needs you to take breaks, because caregivers who never rest become caregivers who burn out, and burned-out caregivers are worse caregivers.

Start small. A two-hour respite. A full afternoon. A Saturday. Build from there. By the time you need a weekend away, you want to have practiced shorter respites so your partner is not experiencing a weekend away as a first-time shock.

Action Challenge

This week, schedule one two-hour respite. Ask a family member, a friend, a neighbor, or a paid helper. Go somewhere that is not your house. Do not do errands. Do something that has nothing to do with caregiving. A walk. A coffee. A movie. Practice the muscle of leaving.

12.5 Support Groups That Actually Help

Not all support groups help. Some make you feel worse. The ones that help share features.

FTD-specific or dementia-specific, not general grief groups. A general grief group may include people whose loss is a distant cousin's death; they cannot hold the weight of your daily life.

Led by a trained facilitator. Good facilitators keep groups from becoming venting pits or advice sessions. They allow room without prescribing.

Regular attendance. Trust builds over time. A group you attend once a month for a year will help more than five different groups over the same period.

Online or in-person, depending on your life. Online groups (such as AFTD's virtual support groups, or UK's Rare Dementia Support groups) are accessible from home, which matters when you cannot leave your partner. In-person groups have a different physical presence that some people prefer.

Separate groups for the well partner vs. the ill partner. If your partner with FTD can still attend a group, their group should be separate from yours. You need to be able to speak freely about the caregiving experience without your partner present.

If a group is not helping, try another. Group fit is real. Do not conclude that support groups do not work based on one bad experience.

12.6 Paid Help And The Math Of Sustainability

At some point, if the disease progresses, paid help becomes non-optional. The math of when and how much to pay is specific to your financial situation, but the principles are universal.

Calculate the true cost of doing it alone. Not only dollars. Your health costs. Your earning capacity if you leave work. The medical bills from caregiver burnout. The long-term costs of your own missed care.

Start earlier than feels necessary. Paying for a few hours of help a week, starting early, is usually sustainable for longer than waiting until you are in crisis and then paying for full-time care.

Use insurance and benefits before personal funds. Long-term care insurance if you have it. VA benefits if your partner served. Medicaid once eligibility is reached. Medicare for the skilled care it does cover.

Hire through agencies, when possible, for liability and reliability. Independent aides can be cheaper and sometimes better, but agencies handle background checks, insurance, taxes, and backup coverage when an aide calls in sick.

Start with tasks, not with your partner. A cleaning service, a meal service, a lawn service, a laundry service. These do not require direct care of your partner and free up hours. Pay for time before you pay for care.

Interview direct-care aides yourself. Vet them. Background checks. References. Training. Ideally, dementia-specific experience. The first few hires may not work out. Do not give up.

Build redundancy. Never rely on one aide or one service. If the aide quits, you should have a backup. Agencies usually provide this; independents usually do not.

The Galvin et al. (2017) figure of $120,000 per year is the true economic cost of FTD caregiving, including both paid services and lost wages. Most families cover a portion of this with Medicaid, family support, and asset drawdown. You will spend money you did not plan to spend. This is one of the cruelties of the disease.

From the Person with FTD's Perspective

Your partner may resist new people coming into the home. This is common in FTD, where changes in routine can produce agitation or anxiety. The resistance is not an argument against help. It is a factor in how help is introduced.

Strategies that help: introduce the aide briefly first, with you present, for non-care tasks. Build familiarity. Use the same aide consistently when possible; rotating strangers is harder than one recurring person. Frame the aide in terms your partner can accept ("Maria is going to help me for a few hours today"). Time respite for when your partner is most settled.

Over time, many people with FTD form attachments to consistent aides that are real and important. The aide is not a substitute for you. They become a supplementary relationship that enriches both lives.

From the Supporting Partner's Perspective

Asking for help, and then accepting it without apologizing, is a skill. Most long-term caregivers did not have this skill at the start. They developed it under duress.

Frances, a year after the produce aisle, said: "I used to think saying no to help was strength. I was wrong. Saying no to help was pride, and pride was going to kill me. Saying yes was the hardest thing I ever did. It was also the only reason I am still here."

You may have to learn to receive before you can receive well. It gets easier. Keep practicing. The team you build this year is the team that carries you through next year.

Practical Strategies and Scripts

When someone says "let me know if I can help": "Actually, yes. I have a list. Can you do item 4? It's picking up the dry cleaning on Friday." Specific. Immediate. Gives them something to say yes to.

When a family member says they are "too busy" to help: "I understand. When you have capacity, here's what would help most. In the meantime, can you call on Saturday? Just call, to check in. That is also help."

When a stranger or acquaintance offers help: "Thank you. I am grateful for the offer. Here's a small thing that would actually help." Small, concrete, easy to deliver. Then thank them visibly. People who are thanked are more likely to help again.

When paid help does not do something the way you would: Let it go if it is not safety-critical. Specify only the things that matter. "Please make sure he takes his medicine at noon" matters. "Please fold the towels the way I fold them" does not.

Reflection Prompts

What is on your Specific Ask List? If you do not have one, what could be the first five items?

Who has offered help in the last year that you declined? Could you go back and accept?

What is one paid service you have been resisting? What is the fear underneath the resistance?

If you collapsed tomorrow, who would step in? Do they know they would? Do they know where the instructions are?

The Quick Version

You cannot do FTD caregiving alone for the full arc. The reasons people resist help (fear of failure, not wanting to burden, not knowing what to ask for, standards, partner resistance, cost) are understandable and solvable. A Specific Ask List on your phone converts vague offers into actual help. An FTD-literate care team includes medical specialists, legal and financial professionals, and paid or volunteer direct care; most families need more than they think. Respite care is clinical necessity, not indulgence. Support groups help when they are FTD-specific, well-facilitated, and attended regularly. Paid help is almost always needed eventually; start earlier and smaller than feels necessary.

Chapter 13. Staying Alive Through Caregiving

Teresa's annual physical was on a Tuesday morning. She did not want to go. She had been caring for her husband Eddie for three years, since his bvFTD diagnosis, and she had been skipping her own medical appointments for most of that time. Eddie's cousin was sitting with him that morning, and Teresa had decided, with effort, that she would finally go.

Her doctor, Dr. Silva, had been her primary care physician for twenty years. Dr. Silva looked at the chart for a long moment before speaking. Teresa had gained thirty-two pounds in three years. Her blood pressure was 164 over 98. Her blood glucose was in the pre-diabetic range. Her cholesterol was elevated. She had not slept more than five hours a night in eighteen months.

Dr. Silva set down the chart. She said, "Teresa. I am going to ask you a question, and I want you to think about it seriously before you answer. If you die before Eddie, what happens to Eddie?"

Teresa blinked. She said, "What?"

"If you die first, what happens to him. Who takes care of him."

Teresa did not answer for a long time. Finally she said, "I don't know."

Dr. Silva said, "Then you are going to change what we do in this room starting today. Because the way you are going now, you are going to die before him, and then no one has a plan."

Teresa cried at the doctor's office. She cried in the car. She went home and told Eddie's cousin, who did not understand what she was saying. She got in the shower and cried more.

That night, she canceled two commitments. She called a therapist the next morning and scheduled her first appointment in four years. She booked a respite weekend for six weeks out. She started walking for twenty minutes every morning, with Eddie, who liked walking.

Four months later, her blood pressure was 128 over 82. She had lost six pounds. She was sleeping seven hours a night. She was still tired. She was no longer depleted.

Dr. Silva looked at the chart at the next visit and said, "You listened."

Teresa said, "I listened because you asked the right question. Nobody had asked me that question before."

Chapter Principle

The caregiver who dies first leaves the person with FTD with no plan, no advocate, no one who remembers who they used to be. You are not being noble by neglecting yourself. You are building a disaster. This chapter is about the specific work of staying alive, awake, and mostly well through a caregiving arc that can last a decade.

13.1 The Caregiver Who Dies First

Research on caregiver mortality is sobering. A landmark study by Schulz and Beach (1999) found that older spousal caregivers who reported caregiving-related mental or emotional strain had mortality risks approximately 63 percent higher than non-caregiving spouses of the same age over a four-year period. Subsequent research has reported that caregiver mortality risk is not uniform across all caregivers and is most elevated among those experiencing high strain, including many spouses caring for people with dementia.

The mechanisms are straightforward. Chronic stress elevates cortisol. Elevated cortisol over years produces hypertension, insulin resistance, weight gain, and immune suppression. Chronic sleep deprivation has the same effects. Delayed or skipped medical care means that treatable problems become untreated problems. Social isolation, common in FTD caregivers, has an independent effect on mortality similar in magnitude to smoking.

The Emma Heming Willis book describes a neurologist telling her, in the early months after Bruce Willis's diagnosis, that caregivers sometimes die before the people they are caring for, because the stress of caregiving is that severe. This is not a rhetorical warning. It is an observation from clinicians who have watched it happen.

The practical implication: your health is not optional. It is infrastructure. You cannot sustain the work of caregiving on a body you are not maintaining. The tasks in this chapter are not indulgences. They are load-bearing.

13.2 Sleep Is A Caregiving Tool

Sleep is the most important and most sacrificed resource in FTD caregiving. A partner who sleeps six hours a night reliably will outperform a partner who sleeps four hours a night inconsistently, at almost every caregiving task, within a week.

The challenges to sleep in FTD caregiving are specific:

Your partner's sleep is disturbed. Many people with FTD, especially in later stages, have altered sleep-wake cycles. They get up at night. They roam. You wake up.

Your own vigilance is elevated. You sleep lightly because some part of you is always on alert.

Bed-sharing becomes difficult or impossible. As the disease progresses, sleeping in the same bed may become unworkable because of restlessness, incontinence, or safety issues.

Your schedule is chaotic. Caregiving tasks scatter across the day and night.

Strategies that work:

Separate sleep spaces when needed. Moving to a separate bedroom is not a failure of the marriage. It is a protection of both your sleep and your partner's. You can still be married and sleep in different rooms. Many couples do this long before they have FTD.

Monitoring systems. A baby monitor or camera can let you sleep more deeply because you will hear your partner if they get up. Bed alarms for people with roaming behaviors can serve the same function.

Paid overnight help in later stages. When your partner needs supervision through the night and you cannot provide it without destroying your own sleep, overnight aides become necessary. This is expensive. It is also sometimes the only way you survive.

Protect sleep as a non-negotiable. Seven hours, minimum, whenever possible. Short naps during the day do not fully substitute.

Sleep hygiene basics. Cool room. No screens in bed. No alcohol within three hours of sleeping. Caffeine only before noon. Your caregiving job is too demanding for sloppy sleep hygiene.

If your sleep is collapsing despite efforts, see a doctor. Insomnia is treatable. Untreated insomnia cascades into every other health problem.

13.3 Movement Nutrition And The Body You Are Ignoring

You have probably been paying less attention to your own body than you used to. This is almost universal among long-term caregivers. It is also reversible.

Movement. You do not need to become an athlete. You need to move. Twenty minutes of walking a day, most days, is enough to significantly reduce cardiovascular risk, improve mood, and protect sleep. Walking with your partner, if they can still walk, is a double benefit: exercise for you, structured activity for them. Caregiver health research has long shown that regular physical activity is associated with reduced depression and improved well-being among dementia caregivers (Schulz & Beach, 1999), and tailored, structured activities for the person with FTD have been associated with reductions in behavioral symptoms (O'Connor et al., 2019).

Nutrition. Caregivers often eat what is fast, not what is fueling. The costs accumulate. You do not need a diet. You need basic fuel: protein at every meal, vegetables daily, some fat, reduced sugar. Meal delivery services, if you can afford them, are often the single best investment in your own health.

Medical appointments. Schedule them. Go to them. Cancel only for actual emergencies, not for caregiving logistics. Your physical, your dental cleanings, your eye appointments, your gynecological or prostate screenings, your mammograms, your colonoscopies. The things you used to do on autopilot that have fallen off.

Alcohol and substance use. Caregiver stress frequently produces increased alcohol use. This is common and dangerous. If you are drinking more than you were, track it. If you cannot cut back, talk to a doctor. Do not let this become the way you cope for a decade.

Action Challenge

Before you finish this chapter, schedule one medical appointment you have been putting off. Dental, physical, eye, whatever it is. Put it in your calendar. Put a backup caregiver in the calendar next to the appointment so you cannot talk yourself out of going.

13.4 The Therapist Who Understands Ambiguous Loss

A therapist who understands ambiguous loss and caregiver grief is one of the single most valuable additions to your support team. Not every therapist understands this. Most therapy training focuses on ordinary grief, depression, anxiety. Ambiguous loss is a specialty.

What to look for:

Familiarity with Pauline Boss's framework. Ask directly. "Are you familiar with ambiguous loss?" A therapist who says "tell me more about that" is not the right fit. A therapist who lights up and says "yes, Pauline Boss's work" is probably worth at least three sessions.

Dementia experience, not only cancer or general illness. Dementia caregiving has specific features. Cancer caregiving, while also hard, is structurally different. A therapist with dementia caregiver experience will understand what you are going through without extensive education from you.

Comfort with the "forbidden" feelings. A therapist who flinches when you say you sometimes wish your partner would die is not the therapist for this. A good therapist will hold the feeling without judging it.

Practical as well as emotional. Pure insight-oriented therapy is less useful here than therapy that combines emotional work with practical problem-solving. You need both.

Finding the right therapist may take two or three tries. This is frustrating and worth the effort. The AFTD website has a directory of therapists familiar with FTD. Your neurologist's social worker may also have referrals.

Do not wait until you are in crisis. Start therapy while you can still engage with it. The therapist you develop a relationship with now is the therapist you can lean on when the hardest things happen later.

13.5 Restorative Rest Helps Both Of You

The phrase *caregiver wellness* has been diluted by marketing into something that sounds optional and indulgent. It is not optional, and the science is specific.

Researchers at the Penn FTD Center, including Lauren Massimo and colleagues, have written extensively about the lived experience of FTD spousal caregivers and have argued for the importance of caregiver self-care, restorative activities, and reduction of caregiver strain (Massimo, Kales, & Kolanowski, 2018). The wider caregiver-health literature consistently links chronic caregiver strain with increased risk of depression and mortality (Schulz & Beach, 1999), which is why protected time for restoration is not a luxury but a clinical priority for the caregiver and, indirectly, for the person they care for.

The mechanism is probably bidirectional. Caregivers who take time for themselves are calmer, more patient, and more effective. People with FTD, who often track the emotional state of their caregiver even when they cannot articulate it, respond to the calmer caregiver with calmer behavior.

The research does not support long expensive retreats or elaborate wellness programs. It supports small, consistent, genuine pleasure.

Examples that have been studied or reported:

Thirty minutes alone in a coffee shop with a book.

A weekly yoga class, gardening session, or hobby.

A walk in a park, preferably somewhere with trees.

A phone call with a friend who knew you before the disease.

Time on a creative project that has nothing to do with caregiving.

A bath with the door locked.

The principle is that the time must be genuinely for you, and must recur reliably, and must be guilt-free. The last element is often the hardest to build.

13.6 Building Moments That Are Only Yours

A specific practice that many long-term caregivers describe is building a small weekly schedule of protected time. Not a whole day off. Not a vacation. Just hours, reliably, that belong to you.

Teresa, six months into her new life after the Dr. Silva appointment, had the following standing commitments:

Tuesday and Thursday mornings, 7:00 to 8:00 a.m., walking alone while Eddie slept.

Wednesday evening, 6:00 to 8:00 p.m., therapy appointment (alternating weeks).

Saturday morning, 9:00 to 12:00, Eddie's cousin came over, Teresa went to a coffee shop and read.

Sunday, 2:00 to 5:00, Teresa's book club, Eddie stayed home with a paid aide.

That is approximately ten hours a week of protected time. It is not a lot. It was, for Teresa, the difference between surviving and collapsing.

The principle is that the time is *scheduled*, not opportunistic. Opportunistic time gets colonized by caregiving emergencies. Scheduled time, on the calendar, defended, attended by other people who are counting on you, is more likely to actually happen.

Build your schedule gradually. Start with one hour a week. Add from there.

From the Person with FTD's Perspective

Your partner, on some level, benefits from your restoration. This is easy to doubt when you are leaving the house and they are frowning. The research suggests otherwise. People with dementia who are cared for by rested, supported caregivers have better behavioral outcomes, fewer hospitalizations, and in some studies, slower functional decline.

Your partner may not be able to articulate gratitude for the time you take. Their brain may not be capable of that articulation. What their brain is doing is tracking your emotional state, your physical presence, your tone of voice. A calmer, rested, nourished caregiver is, to their nervous system, a more reliable environment. This is a gift to both of you.

Do not read your partner's inability to thank you as evidence you should not do the thing. Do it because it is the thing to do.

From the Supporting Partner's Perspective

The hardest part of taking care of yourself during caregiving is not the execution. It is the permission. Most caregivers know what they should be doing. They are not doing it because they feel they do not deserve to, because their partner cannot, because no one is watching, because it feels like a betrayal.

The permission has to come from somewhere. Sometimes it comes from a doctor who asks the right question. Sometimes from an adult child who intervenes. Sometimes from a therapist, a pastor, a support group facilitator. Sometimes, eventually, from yourself.

Teresa, a year after her first Dr. Silva appointment, said: "I had to give myself permission to matter. That sounds melodramatic. It is not. I genuinely did not believe my life mattered as much as Eddie's. It took me a year to believe it did. Once I believed it, everything got easier."

You are allowed to matter. You matter. You are not a secondary character in the story of your partner's illness. You are a person having your own life, inside a situation that is also happening. Live your life.

Practical Strategies and Scripts

When you feel guilty for going to a medical appointment: "I am going because I need to keep being here for my partner. Missing my health is not caring for them. It is setting up a future crisis."

When someone says "you are looking tired": "I am tired. That is accurate. I am working on it." Do not minimize. Accurate reporting is part of being seen.

When a family member criticizes you for taking time for yourself: "My doctor and my therapist are both clear that I need this. I welcome your help in covering so I can go. I do not welcome your criticism for going." Firm, polite, no explanation owed.

When you cannot sleep and it is 3:00 a.m.: Do not lie in bed struggling. Get up. Read something boring in a dim room for twenty minutes. Return to bed. If this is a pattern, see a doctor about sleep.

Reflection Prompts

What is your answer to Dr. Silva's question: if you died tomorrow, what happens to your partner?

What medical appointment have you been skipping? When can you schedule it?

What is the restorative practice you would most benefit from? What is one hour this week you could give to it?

Who is a therapist you might call? If you do not know one, who could refer you?

The Quick Version

Spouses providing high-intensity dementia caregiving have significantly elevated mortality risk. The caregiver who dies first leaves the person with FTD with no plan. Sleep is the most sacrificed resource and the most important; protecting it is a caregiving tool, not a luxury. Movement, nutrition, and medical appointments are non-negotiable. A therapist who understands ambiguous loss is uniquely valuable; look for Pauline Boss familiarity and dementia-specific experience. Research shows restorative caregiver practices benefit not only the caregiver but the person with FTD. Protected weekly time, scheduled and defended, is more likely to actually happen than opportunistic time. You are not a secondary character. Your life matters. Live it.

PART FOUR: THE LONGER PATH

Part Four covers the terrain most partners do not want to think about until they have to. Placement. Late-stage FTD. Hospice. Death. The first year after.

These two chapters are different from the others in tone. They are quieter. They are less about action and more about presence. The decisions covered here are fewer and larger. The practical work does not stop, but the emotional work intensifies.

Read these when you are ready. It is okay to skip them for now and come back. It is also okay to read them early, before you need them, because partners who do the thinking in advance tend to make better decisions in the moments they cannot think.

What is true in both chapters is this: love does not end when caregiving ends. The person you have loved, and lost, and kept loving, is yours. What happens to the love after they die is the work of the rest of your life.

Chapter 14. When Home Cannot Hold Them

Luis had been bathing his wife Elena for eighteen months. She had bvFTD with increasing motor symptoms. She had become, over the last six months, progressively more resistant to care. Most mornings the bath was a negotiation. Some mornings it was a struggle. Luis had learned to time it right, to talk her through it, to pick battles.

On a Thursday in late October, something shifted. Elena resisted the bath harder than she ever had. When Luis tried to help her into the tub, she swung her arm and hit him in the chest. He stepped back, shocked. She swung again and caught his jaw. He fell. He heard a small crunch. He could not stand up immediately.

When he finally got to the emergency room three hours later, the CT scan showed a cracked rib and a hairline fracture in his jaw. The ER physician, a younger woman, looked at his chart, at Elena's diagnosis, at Luis's exhaustion, and said, as gently as she could, "Sir. Have you considered memory care?"

Luis looked at her. He said, "I have considered it every day for a year."

The physician nodded. She did not argue. She said, "You do not have to do this alone. You do not have to do this at all, in your house. There are places that understand this disease. You can still love her. You can still visit her every day. The caregiving is what has to change."

On the drive home, Luis called his daughter. He said, "I think it's time." His daughter, who had been waiting months for this call, said, "I'll come. We'll do it together."

Chapter Principle

Placement is a medical decision, not a moral one. The signs that home is no longer viable are specific and recognizable. Facilities that understand FTD exist and are worth finding. The guilt around placement is universal and unfounded. This chapter is about how to recognize the threshold, how to find the right facility, how to move through the transition, and how to stay married to someone in care.

14.1 The Signs Home Is No Longer Enough

Most caregivers know, long before they admit it, that home is becoming unworkable. The admission is the hardest part. Here are the signs that often mean it is time to seriously consider placement.

Physical safety of the person with FTD. Falls you cannot prevent. Wandering that is escalating. Choking or swallowing difficulties that require skilled observation. Medical complexity (seizures, incontinence, aspiration risk) beyond what you can manage.

Physical safety of the caregiver. Like Luis. Injuries from resistive behavior. Back injuries from transferring. Exhaustion that is producing accidents (forgetting medications, falling asleep while driving).

Behavioral symptoms requiring 24-hour supervision. Roaming through the night. Agitation that cannot be de-escalated. Aggressive behavior that puts you, children, or visitors at risk.

Caregiver health collapse. Hospitalizations. Cardiovascular events. Depression severe enough to impair function. Substance use that is escalating.

Medical complexity. Multiple chronic conditions needing simultaneous management. Frequent hospitalizations. Wound care. Enteral feeding. Ventilation.

The math no longer works. Even with paid help, you cannot cover the hours needed. The cost of 24-hour home care begins to approach or exceed the cost of facility care, and you are still doing the emotional labor alone.

These signs rarely show up one at a time. They accumulate. A threshold is reached. The question is not if you can handle one more week. It is if the current arrangement is sustainable for the next six months.

14.2 Memory Care Built For Alzheimer's And Why It Matters

Most memory care facilities in the United States and the United Kingdom are designed around the needs of people with Alzheimer's disease. This matters for FTD families, because FTD residents often present differently.

The typical Alzheimer's memory care resident is in their late seventies or eighties, physically frail, with memory impairment as the dominant feature, and with behavioral symptoms that are often responsive to redirection and environmental cues. The facility is designed around this profile: slower pace, memory-based activities, quiet environments, gentle redirection.

The typical FTD resident, especially in the middle stages, may be in their fifties or sixties, physically robust, still mobile, with behavioral symptoms that are more driven by disinhibition, compulsion, and apathy than by memory loss. A standard Alzheimer's memory care unit may not know what to do with a resident who walks fifteen miles a day, who eats other residents' food, who speaks inappropriately to staff, who shows no memory deficit on intake screening.

When touring facilities, ask specifically:

Have you had FTD residents before? How many? What variants?

How do you manage roaming behavior that is purposeful rather than disoriented?

What is your ratio of staff to residents, particularly in the afternoons and evenings?

How do you handle residents who are much younger than your average?

What is your approach to disinhibited behavior that affects other residents or staff?

What specialized training does your staff have in FTD?

What is your policy on hospice? Do you work with hospice agencies that understand FTD?

A facility that has not had FTD residents before is not automatically a bad choice. A facility that has never heard of FTD is a red flag. Look for places where the administrator has at least heard of the disease, and where the nursing director is willing to learn.

Some specialized dementia-care programs, including some assisted living facilities and some skilled nursing facilities, have dedicated FTD-aware units or staff. These are rare. If one exists within a reasonable distance, it is worth the drive.

14.3 The Guilt That Is Not Actually Yours

Placement produces a specific, nearly universal guilt. The form of the guilt varies. The content is the same: *I should be able to do this at home. I promised. I failed.*

The promises made before an FTD diagnosis often include some version of "I will never put you in a home." Many partners remember making this promise, sometimes decades earlier. They hold themselves to it against evidence that keeping the promise is destroying them both.

Consider the promise more carefully. When your partner said, "please don't ever put me in a home," they were imagining a scenario where they could be cared for at home without harming you. They were not imagining a scenario where keeping them at home meant you dying of a stress-related heart attack while they roamed the neighborhood at 3 a.m. If you had asked them, at the time, "what if keeping you at home means destroying my health?" the answer most people give is, "then find a place where I can be cared for safely."

The promise you made was not a promise to sacrifice yourself. It was a promise to care for them well. Sometimes caring for them well means finding a facility that can do what you cannot.

The guilt, once the decision is made, often transforms. It does not disappear. It shifts from "I am failing my partner" to "I am handling an impossible situation as well as I can." The first framing paralyzes. The second one allows action.

Luis, three months after Elena moved to a memory care facility, said: "I thought I was abandoning her. I was not. I was finding her a place where she could be cared for by multiple people around the clock, which was never going to be possible in our house. I visit her every day. She is calmer than she was at home. I am not injured anymore. We are both better off. The guilt told me this would be worse. The guilt was wrong."

14.4 How To Tour A Facility

When you tour facilities, tour at least three. Tour with your eyes open. Tour twice when possible, once scheduled and once unscheduled.

What to notice on the scheduled tour. The smell. A clean facility smells like cleaning products. A neglected facility smells like urine. Ask yourself how the residents you see are being treated. Are staff interacting with residents, or ignoring them? Are residents dressed, groomed, engaged? Are call lights being answered? Are dining rooms clean? Are bathrooms clean?

What to notice on the unscheduled tour. Drop in at an inconvenient time. A Saturday afternoon, a weekday dinner, an evening after 8 p.m. This tells you what staffing and care are like when no one is performing for visitors. A facility that is well-run at 2 p.m. on a Wednesday and poorly staffed at 7 p.m. on a Saturday is not as well-run as the first tour suggested.

Talk to other families. Most administrators will offer you references. Ask to speak with current residents' family members. Ask specifically about FTD if the facility has had FTD residents. Ask what has been hard and what has been good. No facility is perfect.

Check regulatory records. In the US, Medicare's Nursing Home Compare and state inspection reports are public. Recent citations for abuse, neglect, or medication errors matter. A perfect record is rare; a pattern of violations is a red flag.

Understand the contract. Level of care fees. Escalation schedules. What triggers a move to a higher level of care. Discharge criteria (can they ask your partner to leave, and for what reasons?). End-of-life policies.

Trust your gut. You will walk into some facilities and feel something off. You will walk into others and feel at ease. Your gut is picking up on things you cannot articulate. Take the gut seriously.

Action Challenge

If you have not toured a facility yet, schedule one tour this month, even if you are years from needing placement. Knowing what is available, and having a relationship with one or two facilities you like, makes the decision in crisis dramatically easier.

14.5 Paying For Long-Term Care

Memory care costs in the United States in 2025 range from $6,000 to $12,000 per month, depending on region and level of care. Specialized dementia care, particularly for younger residents or residents with complex needs, can run higher. In the United Kingdom, costs vary by region and type of care, but are similarly substantial.

Sources of payment, layered:

Long-term care insurance. If your partner purchased a policy before diagnosis. Check the policy carefully. Elimination periods, daily benefits, and care settings covered vary. Most policies are sold as part of a broader financial plan, which means you may have forgotten you had one.

Veterans benefits. If your partner is a veteran, Aid and Attendance benefits can help with assisted living or memory care costs. Work with an accredited Veterans Service Officer. The VA is underutilized; many eligible veterans never apply.

Medicaid. Covers long-term care in most states after spend-down. Rules vary by state. Start planning years in advance, because the Medicaid look-back period (five years in most states) penalizes asset transfers made close to application.

Medicare. Does not cover long-term custodial care. Covers short-term skilled nursing after a qualifying hospitalization. This limitation is the most misunderstood element of American elder care financing.

Personal funds. Savings. Home equity. Retirement accounts. Most families deplete these.

Family contributions. Sometimes adult children contribute, especially in blended families or where children have capacity and willingness.

An elder law attorney is worth the money at this stage. Asset protection strategies, executed early and legally, can make the difference between depletion and sustained financial stability. Medicaid planning is not a loophole. It is a legal and ethical framework that exists precisely because American healthcare financing assumes families will be destroyed by long-term care costs, and the law allows certain protections.

14.6 Staying Married To Someone In Care

Placement changes the shape of the marriage, not its existence. Your partner lives in a facility. You live at home. You are still married.

Practices that help:

Visit on a schedule. Every day, every other day, three times a week. Whatever fits. The schedule matters more than the frequency. Predictability helps both of you.

Stay involved in care. Attend care plan meetings. Know the staff. Build relationships with the nurses and aides who are with your partner most. These people are the daily presence in your partner's life now. Treat them as partners in care.

Bring home into the facility. Photos. A favorite blanket. Familiar music. Smells from home. These turn an institutional room into a place that still holds some of your shared life.

Advocate. You are still the translator. You know what your partner needs that they cannot ask for. Speak up when something is wrong. Do it firmly and respectfully.

Let the marriage change shape. The content of your visits will change. Early after placement, you may spend visits talking, walking, holding hands. Later, you may sit in silence and hold their hand. Later still, you may simply be present while they sleep. All of this is the marriage.

Build a life outside the facility. Placement often, paradoxically, frees up capacity to rebuild parts of your own life that had been lost to caregiving. Some partners return to work. Some reconnect with friendships. Some develop new hobbies. This is not betrayal. Your partner needs you to be a functioning human who visits, not a depleted one who sits vigil.

From the Person with FTD's Perspective

Your partner, moving into a facility, may not understand what is happening in the way you would expect. Depending on the stage, they may not recognize the move as significant. They may ask to go home for weeks afterward. They may adjust to the new environment faster than you.

The adjustment period, according to most facility staff, is roughly two to six weeks. After that, routines take hold. Your partner's brain, which was struggling to cope with the unpredictability of home, often responds well to the structure and consistency of a good facility.

Distressing behaviors in the first weeks are common. These usually resolve. If they do not, the facility may not be the right fit, or your partner may need medication adjustments. Work with the care team.

What does not go away, typically, is your partner's recognition of you. They may not know your name. They may not know the facility is not their home. They will, in most cases, know you are someone important. The face-recognition and relational-warmth circuitry often persists longer than other cognitive functions.

From the Supporting Partner's Perspective

You will cry in the parking lot after the first few visits. This is normal. You will feel, at times, that you have abandoned your partner. This is the guilt talking. It is not the truth.

Luis, six months after Elena moved to her facility, said: "The hardest day of my life was the day I admitted her. The easiest day of my life was the day, six weeks later, when I realized she was doing better than she had been at home, and I was doing better than I had been at home, and we were both still together, just in a different shape. I wish someone had told me it would look like that."

Not every placement story is like Luis's. Some facilities fail. Some partners adjust poorly. But many families find, looking back, that placement was the decision that allowed both partners to survive the last chapter of the disease with some dignity and connection intact.

Practical Strategies and Scripts

When a family member disagrees with placement: "I have thought about this more than you can know. I have consulted with my partner's neurologist and my own doctor. This is the decision. I welcome your help in the transition. I do not welcome debate about the call itself."

When you visit and your partner does not recognize you: Do not correct. Do not ask "do you know who I am?" Enter the room warmly. Use your name. "Hi, it's Luis. I brought you some of those crackers you like." Recognition is not the test of the visit. Presence is.

When a staff member describes a difficult behavior and blames your partner: "He has frontotemporal dementia. He cannot choose those behaviors. Let's talk about what we can change in his environment or routine to reduce them." Redirect toward environmental modification.

When you feel guilty after a visit: Go home. Eat something. Rest. The guilt is grief in a different shape. It does not tell you if you made the right decision. You made a decision you thought through. Trust yourself.

Reflection Prompts

Where are you in the cascade of signs that home is becoming unworkable? What would have to change for placement to be necessary?

If you have not toured facilities, what has stopped you? What would make it easier to start?

What promise, made years ago, is still operating in your thinking? Does it need to be renegotiated with the person you made it to, if that is still possible?

What would your marriage look like, with your partner in care? What parts of it do you want to preserve?

The Quick Version

Placement is a medical decision, not a moral one. The signs that home is no longer viable accumulate rather than arriving at once; they include physical safety of both partners, behavioral symptoms requiring 24-hour supervision, caregiver health collapse, and math that no longer works. Most memory care facilities are designed for Alzheimer's; FTD residents often present differently, and finding an

FTD-aware facility makes the transition dramatically easier. Guilt around placement is nearly universal and largely unfounded; the promise you made was to care for your partner well, not to sacrifice yourself. Tour at least three facilities, at least twice each. Paying for long-term care is a layered problem requiring long-term care insurance, VA benefits where applicable, Medicaid planning, and personal funds; an elder law attorney is worth the money. Marriage continues in a new shape after placement. Visit on a schedule, bring home into the facility, and build a life outside it.

Chapter 15. Comfort Care and Saying Goodbye

Anita sat beside her husband Dev in the hospice suite. Dev had not spoken in eleven months. He could no longer walk. He was on comfort-focused care. He breathed. He slept. He sometimes opened his eyes and looked at the ceiling.

It was a Tuesday afternoon in March. An aide named Rosa came in to reposition him. Rosa hummed while she worked. She hummed a Beatles song, "Here Comes the Sun." Anita had not heard the song in years. Rosa was gentle with Dev. She moved him carefully. She said, to him, as she worked, "You're doing great, Dev. That's it. Okay, love, let's get your other side."

As Rosa hummed, Dev's hand, which had been still for months, lifted, very slightly, off the sheet. His fingers moved. Just a little. Just a few seconds. Then his hand settled back down.

Anita watched this happen. She felt something she had not felt in a long time, something that was not exactly grief and not exactly joy, but some third thing she did not have a name for. Rosa saw it too. She smiled at Anita. She said, "He's still in there. Music reaches him. It always does."

Anita cried quietly, sitting in the chair. Dev died twelve days later, peacefully, in the early hours of a Saturday morning, while Anita held his hand.

At the funeral, Anita did not know how to feel. She had been grieving Dev for eight years. She had been grieving him more intensely for the last two. His death was, in some ways, a relief. It was also the end of a marriage of forty-one years. She had been two people, wife and caregiver, for almost a decade. Now she was a widow. She did not know, yet, who a widow was.

Chapter Principle

Late-stage FTD and the death itself are often, for the partner, less shocking than the long years of ambiguous loss that preceded them. What can be shocking is the bereavement after, which is grief on top of grief, and the reconstruction of a self that has been subsumed into caregiving. This chapter is about the last months, the hospice decision, the death, and the first year after.

15.1 What Late-Stage FTD Looks Like

Late-stage FTD varies by subtype and by individual. Across studies, median survival from diagnosis ranges from approximately three years for some subtypes to nine or more years for semantic variant FTD, with most deaths attributable to end-stage features such as immobility, dysphagia and aspiration, and infection. There are common patterns.

Mobility declines. Walking becomes unsteady, then assisted, then impossible. Falls become frequent. Transfers require two people. Eventually your partner is bed-bound.

Swallowing becomes impaired. Choking episodes increase. Aspiration risk rises. Eating becomes slower, then pureed, then sometimes discontinued.

Incontinence becomes persistent. Bladder first, often, then bowel. Full-time adult diapering.

Communication, in many cases, ceases entirely. Your partner stops speaking. They may stop making eye contact, or do so rarely. In bvFTD, the flattening that started earlier deepens. In PPA, the language that had been progressively lost is now entirely lost.

Sleep changes. More time spent asleep. Less clear distinction between sleep and wake.

Weight loss. Progressive, often substantial. Many people with late FTD become quite thin despite any efforts to maintain weight.

Medical complications. Aspiration pneumonia. Urinary tract infections. Pressure ulcers. Seizures in some cases. These become the common causes of death.

The trajectory at this stage is typically measured in months, not years. Life expectancy from symptom onset in FTD averages 8 to 10 years, but by the time your partner is bed-bound, mute, and medically complex, the time frame has shortened considerably.

None of this should be shocking if you have been paying attention. It is still hard.

15.2 Why Hospice Criteria Fail FTD Families

Hospice care in the United States is governed by Medicare rules that require a six-month prognosis, as certified by two physicians, for eligibility. For Alzheimer's disease, there are specific functional criteria that have been validated. For FTD, there are not.

The result is a specific and recurring problem for FTD families. Your partner may be dying. They may be bed-bound, mute, and cognitively absent. They may still, on some standardized scale, not meet the Alzheimer's-calibrated hospice criteria, because FTD presents differently from Alzheimer's. They may be younger and physically more robust than the typical Alzheimer's hospice patient. They may have better preserved memory (because FTD spares memory until late). They may be judged ineligible for hospice when they clearly need it (Association for Frontotemporal Degeneration, n.d.).

Advocating for hospice enrollment for a person with FTD often requires:

A neurologist letter specifically addressing FTD prognosis and why standard criteria do not apply.

Documentation of functional decline in FTD-specific terms (loss of language, loss of independent eating, loss of independent mobility, incontinence, pneumonia, weight loss).

Choosing a hospice agency with FTD experience. Not all agencies are equally willing to enroll FTD patients. AFTD maintains guidance and referrals.

Persistence. Some families are denied initially and approved on appeal. Do not accept a single denial as final.

Escalation. If your agency will not enroll, try another. Quality varies. A hospice that will not take your partner is not the only hospice in your area.

Palliative care is not the same as hospice and is often easier to access. Palliative care focuses on symptom management and quality of life without the prognosis requirement. Many hospitals and clinics have palliative care services. If hospice is not yet available, palliative care can bridge the gap.

15.3 Advocating For Comfort Care

At some point, the goals of care shift. Earlier in the disease, goals might include slowing progression, optimizing function, managing behavioral symptoms. At some point, these goals no longer apply. Your partner is not going to recover. Function is not going to improve. The goal becomes comfort.

Comfort care, also called comfort-focused care or aggressive symptom management, means:

Treating pain and discomfort proactively. Many people in late-stage FTD cannot articulate pain. Trained staff use behavioral signs (grimacing, restlessness, guarding, vocal sounds) to identify pain and treat it.

Skin care. Preventing and treating pressure ulcers. Repositioning. Specialized mattresses.

Bowel and bladder care. Dignified, regular, attentive.

Oral care. Regular swabbing to prevent dry mouth and oral infections, especially if eating has slowed or stopped.

Presence and touch. Even when language is gone, the person often responds to gentle presence.

Not treating reversible problems aggressively if they would prolong suffering without meaningful life extension. This is the decision family members often agonize over. An aspiration pneumonia could be treated with IV antibiotics in a hospital, possibly extending life by weeks or months, with the person returning to the same declining trajectory. Or it could be treated for comfort at home with oral antibiotics or none at all, with the understanding that this infection may be the one that ends the disease.

Advance directives drafted earlier in the disease become operative here. If your partner expressed, while they had capacity, wishes about comfort care over life extension, those wishes should guide decisions now. If they did not, you become the decision-maker, and you are allowed to make the decision based on what you believe they would have wanted.

The medical system is not always aligned with comfort goals. Some physicians default to aggressive intervention. You may need to advocate, repeatedly, for a comfort-focused approach. A palliative care physician or hospice team can be your ally in this advocacy.

15.4 The Last Weeks And What To Expect

The last weeks of FTD, like the last weeks of any long illness, have predictable features, even as the specific timeline varies.

Reduced intake. Your partner eats and drinks less. The body is preparing. Do not force feeding. This is often distressing to family members who have been focused on nutrition for years. Trust the body. Offer food and fluid as comfort, not as obligation.

More time asleep. Periods of alertness become shorter and less frequent.

Changes in breathing. Periods of rapid breathing, periods of slower breathing, sometimes periods without breathing for several seconds (apnea). This is called Cheyne-Stokes respiration. It is not distressing to the person. It is distressing to family members who do not know what it is. Ask the hospice nurse to explain it to you.

"Death rattle." A gurgling sound caused by secretions in the throat when the person can no longer swallow or cough. This is almost never distressing to the person. It is very distressing to families. Positioning and, if needed, medication can reduce it.

Periods of apparent lucidity. Many dying people have brief, sometimes surprising, periods where they seem more present than they have been in months. These often happen hours to days before death. They are gifts. They are not reversal of the dying process.

Changes in skin color. Mottling, especially of the extremities, as circulation slows.

The actual death. Usually peaceful, especially with good hospice care. Breath slows. Pauses lengthen. Eventually a pause does not end.

Be present if you can. Do not feel obligated to be there every moment. Many people die in the brief window when family has stepped out. This is common enough that some dying people seem, in some way, to choose it. Do not read meaning into the timing of your presence or absence.

After death, there is no hurry. Sit with your partner. Take as much time as you need. If hospice is involved, they will guide the next steps. If not, the funeral home will come when you call.

15.5 Brain Donation As A Gift To Research

FTD research depends on post-mortem brain tissue. The disease can only be definitively diagnosed at autopsy, and ongoing research into causes, mechanisms, and treatments requires donated brain tissue from FTD patients.

AFTD coordinates a brain donation program in partnership with the Mayo Clinic and several other centers. The process needs to be set up in advance, ideally months before death, because it requires coordination between hospice, funeral home, and the research center. A brain-only donation does not interfere with an open-casket funeral. It is typically completed within hours of death.

The decision to donate is a family decision. Some families find meaning in it as a gift to future patients. Some do not. Both choices are legitimate.

If you are considering it:

Contact AFTD (theaftd.org) or UCSF, UPenn, Mayo, or another research center.

Complete paperwork while your partner has capacity, if possible, or you have POA.

Coordinate with hospice so they know the plan.

Inform the funeral home in advance.

Families who have donated often describe it as one of the few moments in the disease where they felt they could take an action that had meaning beyond their own family. The gift is real. The choice is yours.

Action Challenge

If you have not discussed brain donation with your partner (if they still have capacity) or with your family, have the conversation. It is not morbid. It is planning. It is also time-sensitive, because the donation requires advance arrangement.

15.6 The First Year After

Bereavement after a long illness, and particularly after FTD, is different from acute bereavement.

You have been grieving for years. You expect to be done, or further along, or to feel some kind of relief that the anticipated ending has come. Many people feel something like this in the first days and weeks. It is sometimes called *delayed emotional release* or, more pessimistically, *survivor guilt*.

Then, often around two to four months in, something else arrives. You realize you are grieving again, and differently. The person is definitively gone. There is no more caregiving, which is itself a loss (the structure of your days has disappeared). The social identity of caregiver-spouse is gone too, and what replaces it is unclear.

This second wave of grief often surprises partners. They thought they had done the grief. They had done a lot of grief. They had not done all of it.

What helps, in the first year:

Do not make major decisions for the first six to twelve months. Selling the house, moving cities, new relationships. Widowed people who make big decisions in the first year often regret them.

Let the caregiver identity detach slowly. You were a caregiver for years. That identity does not evaporate. Friendships formed through caregiving, skills developed, routines built, all of these are still yours. They just no longer have their original object.

Expect physical effects. The year after losing a long-illness spouse is a higher-risk year for physical illness in the survivor. The widowhood effect is real. Take care of yourself deliberately.

Seek grief support specific to dementia bereavement. Groups and therapists familiar with this specific kind of grief exist. AFTD and the Alzheimer's Association both run bereavement groups.

Allow ambivalence. You will feel relief. You will feel guilt about the relief. You will feel love. You will feel freedom. You will feel loss. All of these can be true at once. None cancels any of the others.

Find ways to carry the person forward. Photographs. Stories told to grandchildren. A charitable donation in their name. Advocacy work for FTD. The love does not die with them. It needs, over time, somewhere to go.

15.7 Who You Are Now

At some point in the first or second year, usually unpredictably, you will have a new experience: a moment of feeling fully yourself, not as caregiver, not as widow, just as yourself. The moment is often short. It may not happen at a moment you expected. Many widows and widowers describe the first such moment as happening on a walk, or at a coffee shop, or doing something mundane.

The moment matters because it is evidence that the self you were afraid was lost is not lost. It was buried. Caregiving buries a lot of the self. Bereavement uncovers pieces, slowly.

Who you are now is someone who has loved a person through a catastrophic disease. That experience is in you. It has changed you. The change is not erasable. It is also not the whole of who you are.

Many people who have done this work find that it leads them somewhere new. Some become advocates. Some start foundations. Some go back to work in new fields. Some become volunteers at hospice, or in dementia support groups, or in research programs. Some simply live their lives with a new depth of understanding about what matters and what does not.

Anita, eighteen months after Dev died, started volunteering at the hospice where he had died. She sat with other dying patients. She held hands. She hummed Beatles songs. She said, to one patient who could not respond, "You're doing great, love. That's it."

She said, later, to a friend: "I thought the caregiving was over. It is not over. I am doing it for other people now. The love had to go somewhere. I put it here. It feels like what he would have wanted, if he could still want things."

Whatever you do with what the disease has given you, whatever shape your life takes now, you are still the person who did this work. The love you gave was real. The loss you have carried is real. The life you have left is yours.

From the Person with FTD's Perspective

In the last weeks of FTD, your partner may not appear to be experiencing anything at all. This is not necessarily the case. Research on consciousness in late-stage dementia suggests that some awareness may persist even when overt responsiveness is absent. Your partner may hear you. They may sense your presence.

They may, on some level below articulation, know they are not alone.

Act as if they know. Not because we are certain they do, but because behaving as if they do is better for both of you than the alternative. Speak gently. Play familiar music. Hold their hand. Say what needs to be said. If they cannot hear you, it costs you nothing. If they can hear you, it is everything.

From the Supporting Partner's Perspective

You will, in the hours or days after the death, experience something unusual. You will be exhausted in a way you did not know was possible, and also, in some strange way, calm. The emergency has ended. Your body may take weeks to understand this. You may sleep more than you have in years. You may not know what to do with your hands.

Anita, three weeks after Dev's death, said: "I kept picking up my phone to check on him. He was not there to check on. I had to retrain my whole nervous system. I didn't know how much of my body was always listening for him until he was no longer there to listen for."

Give yourself time. Do not rush. The structure you built, the routines, the vigilance, the readiness for crisis, all of it is still in your body. It will take months for your body to believe the emergency is over. That is normal. You are not broken. You are recovering from a very long watch.

Practical Strategies and Scripts

When a physician recommends aggressive intervention that does not align with comfort goals: "We have a comfort-focused care plan in place. My partner has an advance directive specifying comfort over extension. I am the healthcare POA. Please document that we are declining [intervention]."

When family members disagree about end-of-life care: "I understand this is hard. My partner's expressed wishes, documented in the advance directive, are what guides our decisions. I am happy to share the document with you. I am not going to change the plan based on disagreement."

When someone asks how you are in the first months after the death: "I'm okay. It's strange. I grieved so much already, and now I'm grieving again differently. Thank you for asking." Accurate. Brief. Not bright. Not bottomless.

When you find yourself still listening for your partner weeks after the death: Do not push it away. Acknowledge it. "I was listening for him just now. He is not here to listen for." Say it gently. The body will eventually learn.

Reflection Prompts

What does comfort care mean in your partner's case? Have the documents and conversations been had?

What would a good death look like for your partner, and for you? What do you want to be in place?

What will you do in the first month after your partner dies? Not for them. For you. Who will be with you? Where will you be?

What do you want to carry forward from this experience? What is the love going to do when your partner is no longer there to give it to?

The Quick Version

Late-stage FTD has recognizable features: reduced mobility, impaired swallowing, incontinence, cessation of communication, increased sleep, weight loss, and medical complications. Hospice criteria are calibrated for Alzheimer's and frequently fail FTD families; advocacy is often required for enrollment. Comfort care shifts goals from disease management to dignity and symptom relief. The last weeks have predictable features that are easier to face when you know what to expect. Brain donation is a meaningful option that requires advance arrangement. The first year after includes a second wave of grief that often surprises partners who thought they had grieved already. Major decisions should wait six to twelve months. Who you are now includes everything you did, and also more than caregiving. The love you built has to go somewhere. Where it goes is up to you.

A Letter to the Person Holding This Book

You picked up this book because someone you love has frontotemporal dementia, or because you suspect they do, or because a doctor said words last week that rearranged your life.

I do not know your name or your story. I know a few things about you anyway.

You are tired. You have been tired for longer than you can remember. You are carrying something that most of the people around you do not understand, and you have stopped trying to explain it because explaining takes energy you do not have.

You love someone whose brain is changing in ways that make them harder to love, and you love them anyway, and the gap between those two facts is where you live now.

You did not choose this. You are doing it anyway.

This book was written to be the book that should have been handed to you in the neurologist's parking lot, or the book that should have been on the shelf when you first typed "why is my husband acting strange" into a search engine at 2 a.m. It is not a memoir. It is not a textbook. It is a practical guide for the person sleeping next to someone whose personality is disappearing, written by someone who believes you deserve better than a pamphlet and a follow-up in three months.

You will not use every chapter. Some chapters are for partners of people with behavioral variant FTD. Some are for partners of people with primary progressive aphasia. Some are for both. Read what you need. Skip what you do not. Come back when something changes.

Three things I want you to carry out of this book, if you carry nothing else:

The behaviors are the disease, not the person. This reframe will save your sanity on the hardest days.

You cannot do this alone, and trying to will break you. Build the team. Accept the help. Schedule the respite. Your partner needs you alive more than they need you heroic.

Your life still matters. Not only as a vehicle for caregiving. Your life, your health, your friendships, your sleep, your pleasure. These are not extras. They are the infrastructure that makes everything else possible.

You are doing something almost nobody around you can fully understand. You are doing it with less support than you deserve. You are still here, still reading, still trying.

That is not small. That is everything.

With respect and without platitudes,

Quick-Reference Appendix

This appendix contains four tools you can photocopy, screenshot, or tear out and keep on your refrigerator. They are designed to be used, not admired.

Appendix A. FTD Awareness Card Template

Print on card stock. Cut to wallet size. Keep five copies: one in your partner's wallet, one in each jacket pocket, one in your wallet, one in the car.

Front of card:

MY NAME IS: ____

I HAVE FRONTOTEMPORAL DEMENTIA

This is a brain disease that can affect my behavior, speech, and judgment. I may say or do things that seem inappropriate. I am not intoxicated, dangerous, or being rude on purpose.

Please be patient. Please call my emergency contact.

EMERGENCY CONTACT: ____

PHONE: ____

Back of card:

DIAGNOSIS: ____

(e.g., bvFTD, semantic variant PPA, nfvPPA)

NEUROLOGIST: ____

NEUROLOGIST PHONE:
____

MEDICATIONS:
____

ALLERGIES:
____

For more information: theaftd.org

Appendix B. Behavior Log Template

Use this log to document changes over time. Bring it to every neurology appointment. The more specific and dated the entries, the more useful they are.

Instructions: Record one entry per incident. Be concrete. Use exact quotes when possible. Describe what you observed, not what you interpreted.

Date	Time	What happened (exact behavior, quote, or action)	Setting and context	Your partner's response when addressed	Notes

Tips for a strong log:

Write entries within 24 hours of the incident. Memory fades fast under stress.

Use specific language. "Said something rude" is less useful than "told the server her accent was hard to listen to."

Note what is different from your partner's baseline. "Never would have done this before 2023" is valuable context.

Record the frequency. "Third time this month" matters more than a single event.

Do not editorialize in the log itself. Save your interpretation for the appointment.

Appendix C. Ten-Task Help List Template

Keep this list on your phone. When someone says "let me know if I can help," read them three items and let them choose one. Update the list weekly.

Instructions: Fill in ten specific, concrete, two-hour tasks that someone could do to help you this week. Replace completed items with new ones.

1. ____
2. ____
3. ____
4. ____
5. ____
6. ____
7. ____

8.

_______________________________\
____

9.

_______________________________\
____

10.

_______________________________\
____

Starter ideas if you are drawing a blank:

Sit with my partner for two hours so I can leave the house.

Pick up groceries from this list.

Drive my partner to an appointment.

Bring dinner on a specific night.

Mow the lawn or shovel the walk.

Walk the dog.

Do one load of laundry.

Sit with my partner Saturday morning so I can go to a support group.

Take my car for an oil change.

Come over and do any one task from the kitchen whiteboard without asking.

Appendix D. Conversation Scripts by Chapter

These scripts are pulled from Chapters 1 through 15. They are meant to be adapted, not memorized. Use them as starting points.

Scripts from Chapter 1. When Something Feels Wrong

If your partner's doctor dismisses your concerns:

"I hear you that a lot of this can look like depression or stress. I would like to rule out a neurological cause before we try an antidepressant. Can you refer us to a memory clinic or behavioral neurologist for evaluation?"

If your partner refuses the appointment:

"The kids would feel better if we both got checkups this year. I made us both appointments. I'll go first."

If a family member accuses you of exaggerating:

"I don't need you to believe me about the diagnosis. I need you to stop telling me I'm imagining it. We'll know more after the next appointment."

If you need to describe what you are seeing to a doctor in under two minutes:

"Over the past [time frame], I have observed specific, uncharacteristic changes in my spouse's behavior, including [three concrete examples]. These are out of character and have been getting more frequent. I am concerned about an underlying medical cause."

Scripts from Chapter 2. What the FTD Brain Is Doing

When a relative calls it Alzheimer's:

"It's actually called frontotemporal dementia. It's different from Alzheimer's. Memory isn't the main thing. The main thing is personality and behavior."

When explaining the diagnosis to a doctor who has never seen FTD:

"My partner has [bvFTD / svPPA / nfvPPA / lvPPA]. The main features are [behavioral disinhibition / word-meaning loss / effortful speech / word-finding difficulty]. They are cognitively [preserved / affected] in terms of memory. I can send you an AFTD provider info sheet."

Scripts from Chapter 3. The Day Everything Changes

When people ask how you are in the first week:

"We got some hard news. I'm not up to talking about it yet. Thank you for asking."

When someone offers unsolicited advice:

"Thank you. I'm not at a point where I can absorb suggestions yet. I'll come back to you when I am."

When your partner seems unaffected by the diagnosis:

Do not try to make them feel something. The absence of a strong response is often a symptom of the disease itself. Love them through the flatness.

Scripts from Chapter 4. Not Them But the Disease

When a family member blames your partner for a behavior:

"That's not him. That's the disease. He would be horrified if he had the insight to see it. I need you to see it the same way."

When you catch yourself about to say something you will regret:

Leave the room. Close a door. Count to ten. Come back when you are not flooded. Repeat as needed.

Scripts from Chapter 5. Living With Personality Changes

When your partner asks about a lockbox on the pantry:

"The doctor wants us to watch your eating for your blood sugar. This makes it easier."

When a family member says "you're too controlling":

"I'm providing the brain functions his brain can no longer provide. The pantry lock is a medical device. I welcome your help if you'd like to spend a day managing the eating without it."

When apathy hits at noon and the day feels wasted:

Lower the expectation. A single activity, accompanied, counts as a full day. Do not measure the day against what you would have done before the diagnosis.

Scripts from Chapter 6. Finding Words That Still Work

In a restaurant, when your partner cannot read the menu:

"They have a chicken dish you liked last time. Want me to order that?"

When a family member on the phone does not know what to do:

Email them a one-page guide: "[Name] has a kind of dementia that affects his language. He can hear you and understand most of what you say. He may not respond in words. Please keep talking to him. Let him know you love him. You can hang up whenever it feels right."

When a stranger treats your partner as incompetent:

"He understands you. He has a speech condition. You can talk to him directly."

Scripts from Chapter 7. Protecting Your Financial Future

When you set up a POA and your partner resists:

"This is what everyone our age does now. The lawyer recommended it for both of us. It doesn't take anything away from you. It just means if something happens to either of us, the other can keep things running."

When the bank representative does not recognize your POA:

"I have a durable power of attorney on file with this bank. Please verify with your back office. I'll wait."

When your partner wants to buy something unreasonable:

Do not argue about the item. Delay. "Let's sleep on it." The impulse often passes by morning.

Scripts from Chapter 8. Keeping Everyone Safe Together

When a family member says you are overreacting to safety concerns:

"The AFTD and the neurologist both recommend these measures. You are welcome to stay with him for a weekend and see the day-to-day. I'd appreciate the break."

When your partner resists wearing the GPS watch:

"The doctor wants us to track your blood pressure with this." Or: "I want to be able to find you if we get separated when we're out together."

When police arrive for a wandering incident:

"Thank you for finding him. He has frontotemporal dementia. Here's a card explaining. Can you help me get him to the car?"

Scripts from Chapter 9. Grieving Someone Still Here

When someone says "but she's still here, you should be grateful":

"I am grateful. And I'm also grieving. Both things are true. I need you to let both things be true."

When you feel relief that your partner is napping and it feels wrong:

Name it to yourself: "I'm relieved he's napping. That's allowed. Relief is not betrayal. It's oxygen."

Scripts from Chapter 10. Love When Everything Shifts

When a friend asks "is the marriage still a marriage?":

"It is different. The shape has changed. It is still the marriage. I am still his wife. He is still my husband. The content has shifted, not the container."

When your partner exhibits disinhibited sexual behavior in public:

Remove your partner from the setting. Apologize briefly. Do not punish or lecture. Discuss medication and behavioral approaches with the neurologist.

Scripts from Chapter 11. Telling Children What Is Happening

For children ages 4 to 7:

"Daddy's brain is sick. It makes him act different sometimes. It's not because he doesn't love you. Doctors are helping him. If you have questions, you can always ask me."

For children ages 8 to 12:

"Dad has a disease called frontotemporal dementia. It changes his brain over time. It's making him act differently and forget words. Doctors cannot cure it. I'll tell you what's happening as it changes. You can ask me anything."

For children ages 13 to 18:

"This is what the disease is. This is what we know. This is what we don't know. I need to know what you need and when you're struggling. You can have your own feelings about this that are different from mine. We're on the same team."

When a relative criticizes you for telling the children:

"The pediatric psychologist and the neurologist both recommended age-appropriate honesty. The research supports it. I appreciate your concern. I have this."

Scripts from Chapter 12. Building Your Support Team

When someone says "let me know if I can help":

"Actually, yes. I have a list. Can you do item 4? It's picking up the dry cleaning on Friday."

When paid help does not do something the way you would:

Let it go if it is not safety-critical. Specify only the things that matter.

Scripts from Chapter 13. Staying Alive Through Caregiving

When you feel guilty for going to a medical appointment:

"I am going because I need to keep being here for my partner. Missing my health is not caring for them. It is setting up a future crisis."

When a family member criticizes you for taking time for yourself:

"My doctor and my therapist are both clear that I need this. I welcome your help in covering so I can go. I do not welcome your criticism for going."

Scripts from Chapter 14. When Home Cannot Hold Them

When a family member disagrees with placement:

"I have thought about this more than you can know. I have consulted with my partner's neurologist and my own doctor. This is the decision. I welcome your help in the transition. I do not welcome debate about the call itself."

When you visit and your partner does not recognize you:

Do not correct. Do not quiz. Enter warmly. Use your name. "Hi, it's [your name]. I brought you some of those crackers you like."

Scripts from Chapter 14. When Staff Describe Difficult Behavior

"He has frontotemporal dementia. He cannot choose those behaviors. Let's talk about what we can change in his environment or routine to reduce them."

Scripts from Chapter 15. Comfort Care and Saying Goodbye

When a physician recommends aggressive intervention that does not align with comfort goals:

"We have a comfort-focused care plan in place. My partner has an advance directive specifying comfort over extension. I am the healthcare POA. Please document that we are declining [intervention]."

When family members disagree about end-of-life care:

"I understand this is hard. My partner's expressed wishes, documented in the advance directive, are what guides our decisions. I am happy to share the document. I am not going to change the plan based on disagreement."

When someone asks how you are after the death:

"I'm okay. It's strange. I grieved so much already, and now I'm grieving again differently. Thank you for asking."

Resources

The following organizations, programs, and services provide information, support, and advocacy for people with FTD and their care partners. This list was current as of the date of publication. Contact information may change. When in doubt, start with AFTD.

United States

Association for Frontotemporal Degeneration (AFTD)

Phone: 1-866-507-7222

Email: info@theaftd.org

Website: theaftd.org

The primary US nonprofit for FTD. Offers a HelpLine staffed by trained specialists, virtual and in-person support groups, educational webinars, the FTD Disorders Registry, and an extensive resource library. Start here.

AFTD HelpLine

Phone: 1-866-507-7222

Available Monday through Friday, with callback and email options. HelpLine staff can connect you with local services, support groups, legal resources, and clinical trial information.

UCSF Memory and Aging Center

San Francisco, California

Website: memory.ucsf.edu

One of the world's leading FTD research and clinical centers. Offers diagnostic evaluations, second opinions, clinical trials, and family support programs. Home of Dr. Bruce Miller's frontotemporal dementia research program.

Penn Frontotemporal Degeneration Center

University of Pennsylvania, Philadelphia

Website: pennftdcenter.org

A leading clinical and research center specializing in all FTD subtypes. Led by Dr. Murray Grossman and Dr. Lauren Massimo. Offers diagnostic evaluations, research enrollment, and caregiver resources.

Mayo Clinic Neurodegenerative Research Group

Jacksonville, Florida and Rochester, Minnesota

Website: mayo.edu

Major FTD research program with clinical evaluations, genetic testing, and clinical trials.

Massachusetts General Hospital FTD Unit

Boston, Massachusetts

Website: massgeneral.org

FTD clinical and research program within the Department of Neurology.

National Institute on Aging (NIA)

Website: nia.nih.gov

Part of the National Institutes of Health. Provides educational materials on all frontotemporal disorders and information on clinical trials through clinicaltrials.gov.

Alzheimer's Association

24/7 Helpline: 1-800-272-3900

Website: alz.org

While focused primarily on Alzheimer's disease, the Alzheimer's Association provides information on FTD, caregiver support groups, and community programs that serve all dementia types.

ClinicalTrials.gov

Website: clinicaltrials.gov

Search "frontotemporal dementia" to find current research studies enrolling participants. Ask your neurologist which trials may be appropriate.

Social Security Compassionate Allowances Program

Website: ssa.gov/compassionateallowances

All FTD disorders are on the Compassionate Allowances list, which expedites SSDI and SSI applications.

National Alliance for Caregiving

Website: caregiving.org

Resources, research, and advocacy for family caregivers across all conditions.

Family Caregiver Alliance

Website: caregiver.org

Based in San Francisco. Provides education, services, research, and advocacy for family caregivers. Pauline Boss's work on ambiguous loss is featured prominently.

United Kingdom

Rare Dementia Support

Website: raredementiasupport.org

Based at University College London. Provides peer support groups, information, and social activities for people affected by rare dementias including FTD, PPA, and posterior cortical atrophy.

Dementia UK

Website: dementiauk.org

Provides Admiral Nurses, specialist dementia nurses who give one-to-one support to families.

Alzheimer's Society (UK)

Website: alzheimers.org.uk

Helpline: 0333 150 3456

Provides information, support, and services for all forms of dementia including FTD.

FTD Talk

Website: ftdtalk.org

UK-based factsheets and resources for people affected by FTD.

National Hospital for Neurology and Neurosurgery

Queen Square, London

UCL Dementia Research Centre. Major FTD clinical and research center in the UK.

Cambridge Centre for Frontotemporal Dementia and Related Disorders

University of Cambridge

Clinical and research program specializing in FTD.

Australia

The Australian FTD Association

Website: theaftd.org.au

Support, education, and advocacy for Australian families affected by FTD.

Dementia Australia

Website: dementia.org.au

Helpline: 1800 100 500

Information and support for all dementia types.

Canada

Alzheimer Society of Canada

Website: alzheimer.ca

Helpline: 1-855-705-4636

Provides information on all dementias including FTD.

International

GENetic Frontotemporal dementia Initiative (GENFI)

Website: genfi.org.uk

An international research study of families with genetic forms of FTD. Enrolls participants across Europe, Canada, and beyond.

Brain Donation

AFTD Brain Donation Coordination Program

Contact AFTD at 1-866-507-7222 for guidance on arranging brain donation. Coordination must be arranged before death. Brain-only donation does not interfere with open-casket funeral arrangements.

Mental Health and Crisis Support

988 Suicide and Crisis Lifeline (US)

Phone: 988

Available 24/7 by phone and text.

Crisis Text Line (US)

Text HOME to 741741.

Samaritans (UK)

Phone: 116 123

Available 24/7.

Glossary of FTD Terms

Plain-language definitions for terms you will encounter in this book, in medical appointments, in research, and in support groups. Arranged alphabetically.

ABC model. A behavioral framework that stands for Antecedent (what happened before), Behavior (what the person did), and Consequence (what happened after). Used to understand and manage challenging behaviors by modifying the antecedent rather than the consequence.

Advance directive. A legal document that describes the medical care a person wants or does not want if they become unable to make decisions for themselves. Includes living wills and healthcare power of attorney.

Ambiguous loss. A term coined by therapist and researcher Pauline Boss for the grief of losing someone who is still physically present but psychologically or emotionally absent. Central to the experience of loving someone with dementia.

Amyotrophic lateral sclerosis (ALS). A neurodegenerative disease that causes progressive muscle weakness and wasting. Also known as Lou Gehrig's disease. Some people with FTD also develop ALS; this is called FTD-ALS.

Anosognosia. The neurological inability to recognize or be aware of one's own disease or symptoms. Common in bvFTD. Different from denial, which is a psychological defense. In anosognosia, the brain regions that would generate self-awareness are damaged.

Anterior temporal lobes. The front portions of the temporal lobes, located on the sides of the head above the ears. Responsible for word meaning, object knowledge, and face recognition. Atrophy here produces the language symptoms of semantic variant PPA.

Anticipatory grief. Grief that begins before the person has died. In FTD, anticipatory grief can last years and involves mourning personality changes, lost roles, and the future that was expected.

Apathy. A neurological reduction in motivation, drive, and initiative. One of the most common and most damaging symptoms in bvFTD. Different from depression in that the person typically does not feel sad.

Apraxia of speech. Difficulty with the motor planning needed to produce speech sounds, even though the muscles are not weak. Common in nonfluent/agrammatic variant PPA. The person knows what they want to say but cannot coordinate the movements to say it.

Atrophy. Shrinkage of brain tissue due to the death of nerve cells. In FTD, atrophy is concentrated in the frontal and anterior temporal lobes and can be seen on MRI.

Augmentative and alternative communication (AAC). Tools and systems that supplement or replace spoken language. Includes picture boards, communication apps, writing, and gesture. Used when speech becomes limited in PPA.

Behavioral variant FTD (bvFTD). The most common form of FTD. Characterized by changes in personality, behavior, judgment, and social conduct. Memory is relatively preserved in early stages.

Brain donation. The donation of brain tissue after death for research purposes. FTD can only be definitively diagnosed by examining brain tissue. Arrangements must be made before death.

C9orf72. The most common gene associated with genetic FTD. A mutation in this gene causes a repeat expansion that leads to FTD, ALS, or both. Inherited in an autosomal dominant pattern, meaning each child of a carrier has a 50 percent chance of inheriting it.

Caregiver burden. The physical, emotional, social, and financial strain experienced by a person providing care for someone with a chronic or terminal illness. Consistently higher in FTD caregivers than in caregivers of other dementias.

Comfort care. Medical care focused on relieving symptoms, reducing pain, and preserving dignity rather than treating or curing the underlying disease. Also called comfort-focused care.

Compassionate Allowances. A program within the Social Security Administration that expedites disability benefit decisions for conditions with obviously severe symptoms. All FTD disorders have been on this list since 2011.

Compulsive behavior. Repetitive actions performed in a driven, ritualistic way. Common in bvFTD. Examples include repeated hand-clapping, walking the same route daily, hoarding objects, or eating the same food at the same time.

Corticobasal syndrome (CBS). A movement disorder that can overlap with FTD. Features include limb rigidity, clumsiness, and difficulty with purposeful movement (apraxia). Caused by degeneration in the cortex and basal ganglia.

Disinhibition. Loss of the brain's impulse-control mechanism. The person says or does things without the internal check that would normally prevent socially inappropriate behavior. A hallmark symptom of bvFTD.

Durable power of attorney. A legal document that gives another person the authority to make decisions on your behalf, and that remains in effect even if you lose mental capacity. Comes in two forms: financial and healthcare.

Empathy loss. Reduced ability to recognize, understand, or respond to the emotions of others. Common in bvFTD. Research suggests it is primarily a loss of cognitive empathy (reading others' feelings) rather than a loss of all emotional capacity.

Executive function. The set of mental processes that include planning, decision-making, problem-solving, impulse control, and the ability to shift between tasks. Controlled primarily by the frontal lobes. Impaired early in bvFTD.

Frontal lobes. The part of the brain behind the forehead. Responsible for judgment, planning, social behavior, empathy, motivation, and impulse control. The primary site of degeneration in bvFTD.

Frontotemporal degeneration (FTD). The umbrella term for all diseases caused by progressive damage to the frontal and temporal lobes of the brain. Includes bvFTD, all PPA subtypes, and FTD with motor symptoms. Also called frontotemporal dementia or frontotemporal lobar degeneration (FTLD).

FTD-ALS. A combined condition in which a person has both FTD and amyotrophic lateral sclerosis. Progresses faster than either condition alone, typically over two to four years.

FUS. Fused in sarcoma protein. One of the three main proteins that can accumulate abnormally in FTD, along with tau and TDP-43. Less common than the other two.

Genetic counselor. A healthcare professional trained to help families understand genetic test results, assess inherited risk, and make informed decisions about testing. Essential when a genetic form of FTD is suspected.

GRN. The progranulin gene. Mutations in GRN are one of the three most common genetic causes of FTD. Inherited in an autosomal dominant pattern.

Hospice care. A form of comfort-focused care for people in the final stage of a terminal illness, typically with a prognosis of six months or less. In the US, covered by Medicare. Provides medical, emotional, and spiritual support for both the patient and the family.

Hyperorality. Increased eating, changes in food preferences (often toward sweets), and sometimes eating of non-food items. A common symptom of bvFTD resulting from damage to brain regions that regulate eating behavior.

Logopenic variant PPA (lvPPA). A subtype of primary progressive aphasia characterized by word-finding difficulty and impaired sentence repetition. Often associated with Alzheimer's-type brain pathology rather than frontotemporal pathology.

MAPT. The microtubule-associated protein tau gene. Mutations in MAPT cause a form of genetic FTD characterized by tau protein buildup. Inherited in an autosomal dominant pattern.

Medicaid. A joint federal-state program in the United States that provides health coverage, including long-term care, for people with limited income and assets. Covers nursing home care and, in many states, home-based care. Requires asset spend-down to qualify.

Medicare. A federal health insurance program in the United States for people 65 and older or those who have been on SSDI for 24 months. Covers hospitalizations, doctor visits, and some skilled nursing care. Does not cover long-term custodial care.

Mental capacity. The legal and medical ability to understand, weigh, and communicate a decision. Capacity is task-specific (a person can have capacity for simple decisions and not for complex ones) and can fluctuate over time.

Nonfluent/agrammatic variant PPA (nfvPPA). A subtype of primary progressive aphasia characterized by effortful, halting speech and loss of grammatical structure. Often associated with apraxia of speech. Understanding of language is relatively preserved early.

Orbitofrontal cortex. The part of the frontal lobe located just above the eye sockets. Plays a key role in impulse control, social behavior, and decision-making. Atrophy here is a primary driver of disinhibition in bvFTD.

Palliative care. Medical care focused on improving quality of life and managing symptoms for people with serious illnesses. Can be provided at any stage of illness, not only at end of life. Different from hospice in that it does not require a six-month prognosis.

PET scan (positron emission tomography). A brain imaging technique that measures metabolic activity. In FTD, PET scans can show areas of reduced brain activity that may not yet be visible as atrophy on MRI.

Primary progressive aphasia (PPA). A group of neurodegenerative conditions in which language is the dominant symptom. Three subtypes: semantic (svPPA), nonfluent/agrammatic (nfvPPA), and logopenic (lvPPA). Often, but not always, caused by frontotemporal degeneration.

Progressive supranuclear palsy (PSP). A neurodegenerative condition that causes difficulty with balance, walking, and eye movements. Can overlap with FTD. Symptoms may resemble Parkinson's disease but typically do not include tremor.

Respite care. Temporary care of a person with FTD by someone other than the primary caregiver, allowing the caregiver time to rest. Can be provided in-home, at an adult day program, or at a residential facility.

Roaming. Repetitive, purposeful walking or driving of familiar routes. Common in bvFTD. Different from wandering (which implies disorientation) in that the person typically knows where they are and follows the same route.

Semantic variant PPA (svPPA). A subtype of primary progressive aphasia characterized by progressive loss of word meaning. Speech remains fluent but becomes increasingly vague. Also associated with loss of knowledge about objects and faces.

SSDI (Social Security Disability Insurance). A US federal program that provides income to people who cannot work due to disability, based on work history. FTD qualifies for expedited processing through the Compassionate Allowances program.

Tau. A protein that normally helps stabilize the internal structure of nerve cells. In some forms of FTD, tau accumulates abnormally, forming clumps that damage and kill brain cells. One of the three main pathological proteins in FTD.

TDP-43. Transactive response DNA-binding protein 43. A protein that accumulates abnormally in many cases of FTD, particularly in bvFTD and semantic variant PPA. One of the three main pathological proteins in FTD.

Temporal lobes. The parts of the brain located on the sides of the head, above and around the ears. The anterior portions are responsible for word meaning, face recognition, and object knowledge. Degeneration here produces the language symptoms of PPA.

Trazodone. An older antidepressant medication sometimes used to manage behavioral symptoms in FTD, including eating behaviors, sleep disturbance, and irritability. One of the few medications with modest evidence supporting its use in FTD.

References

Allen, J., Oyebode, J. R., & Allen, J. (2009). Having a father with young onset dementia: The impact on well-being of young people. *Dementia, 8*(4), 455-480. https://doi.org/10.1177/1471301209349106

Association for Frontotemporal Degeneration. (2024). *Partners in FTD care: Residential care for people with FTD.* https://www.theaftd.org

Association for Frontotemporal Degeneration. (n.d.). *Hospice care and FTD: Partners in FTD care*. https://www.theaftd.org

Bang, J., Spina, S., & Miller, B. L. (2015). Frontotemporal dementia. *The Lancet, 386*(10004), 1672-1682. https://doi.org/10.1016/S0140-6736(15)00461-4

Boss, P. (2011). *Loving someone who has dementia: How to find hope while coping with stress and grief.* Jossey-Bass.

Chiong, W., Hsu, M., Wudka, D., Miller, B. L., & Rosen, H. J. (2014). Financial errors in dementia: Testing a neuroeconomic conceptual framework. *Neurocase, 20*(4), 389-396. https://doi.org/10.1080/13554794.2013.770886

de Vugt, M. E., Riedijk, S. R., Aalten, P., Tibben, A., van Swieten, J. C., & Verhey, F. R. (2006). Impact of behavioural problems on spousal caregivers: A comparison between Alzheimer's disease and frontotemporal dementia. *Dementia and Geriatric Cognitive Disorders, 22*(1), 35-41. https://doi.org/10.1159/000093102

Diehl-Schmid, J., Schmidt, E. M., Nunnemann, S., Riedl, L., Kurz, A., Förstl, H., Wagenpfeil, S., & Cramer, B. (2013). Caregiver burden and needs in frontotemporal dementia. *Journal of Geriatric Psychiatry and Neurology, 26*(4), 221-229. https://doi.org/10.1177/0891988713498467

Galvin, J. E., Howard, D. H., Denny, S. S., Dickinson, S., & Tatton, N. (2017). The social and economic burden of frontotemporal degeneration. *Neurology, 89*(20), 2049-2056. https://doi.org/10.1212/WNL.0000000000004614

Gorno-Tempini, M. L., Hillis, A. E., Weintraub, S., Kertesz, A., Mendez, M., Cappa, S. F., Ogar, J. M., Rohrer, J. D., Black, S., Boeve, B. F., Manes, F., Dronkers, N. F., Vandenberghe, R., Rascovsky, K., Patterson, K., Miller, B. L., Knopman, D. S., Hodges, J. R., Mesulam, M. M., & Grossman, M. (2011). Classification of primary progressive aphasia and its variants. *Neurology, 76*(11), 1006-1014. https://doi.org/10.1212/WNL.0b013e31821103e6

Heming Willis, E. (2025). *The unexpected journey: Finding strength, hope, and yourself on the caregiving path*. Open Field.

Ikeda, M., Brown, J., Holland, A. J., Fukuhara, R., & Hodges, J. R. (2002). Changes in appetite, food preference, and eating habits in frontotemporal dementia and Alzheimer's disease. *Journal of Neurology, Neurosurgery, and Psychiatry, 73*(4), 371-376. https://doi.org/10.1136/jnnp.73.4.371

Kindell, J., Sage, K., & Cruice, M. (2015). Supporting communication in semantic dementia: Clinical consensus from expert practitioners. *Quality in Ageing and Older Adults, 16*(3), 153-164. https://doi.org/10.1108/QAOA-08-2014-0016

Massimo, L., Kales, H. C., & Kolanowski, A. (2018). State of the science: Apathy as a model for investigating behavioral and psychological symptoms in dementia. *Journal of the American Geriatrics Society, 66*(S1), S4-S12. https://doi.org/10.1111/jgs.15343

Mendez, M. F., Chen, A. K., Shapira, J. S., & Miller, B. L. (2005). Acquired sociopathy and frontotemporal dementia. *Dementia and Geriatric Cognitive Disorders, 20*(2-3), 99-104. https://doi.org/10.1159/000086474

Mioshi, E., Bristow, M., Cook, R., & Hodges, J. R. (2009). Factors underlying caregiver stress in frontotemporal dementia patients. *Dementia and Geriatric Cognitive Disorders, 27*(1), 76-81. https://doi.org/10.1159/000193632

Mioshi, E., Foxe, D., Leslie, F., Savage, S., Hsieh, S., Miller, L., Hodges, J. R., & Piguet, O. (2013). The impact of dementia severity on caregiver burden in frontotemporal dementia and Alzheimer disease. *Alzheimer Disease and Associated Disorders, 27*(1), 68-73. https://doi.org/10.1097/WAD.0b013e318247a0bc

Nunnemann, S., Kurz, A., Leucht, S., & Diehl-Schmid, J. (2012). Caregivers of patients with frontotemporal lobar degeneration: A review of burden, problems, needs, and interventions. *International Psychogeriatrics, 24*(9), 1368-1386. https://doi.org/10.1017/S104161021200035X

O'Connor, C. M., Clemson, L., Brodaty, H., Low, L. F., Jeon, Y. H., Gitlin, L. N., Piguet, O., & Mioshi, E. (2019). The tailored activity program (TAP) to address behavioral disturbances in frontotemporal dementia: A feasibility and pilot study. *Disability and Rehabilitation, 41*(3), 299-310. https://doi.org/10.1080/09638288.2017.1387614

Onyike, C. U., & Diehl-Schmid, J. (2013). The epidemiology of frontotemporal dementia. *International Review of Psychiatry, 25*(2), 130-137. https://doi.org/10.3109/09540261.2013.776523

Rankin, K. P., Gorno-Tempini, M. L., Allison, S. C., Stanley, C. M., Glenn, S., Weiner, M. W., & Miller, B. L. (2006). Structural anatomy of empathy in neurodegenerative disease. *Brain, 129*(11), 2945-2956. https://doi.org/10.1093/brain/awl254

Rascovsky, K., Hodges, J. R., Knopman, D., Mendez, M. F., Kramer, J. H., Neuhaus, J., van Swieten, J. C., Seelaar, H., Dopper, E. G. P., Onyike, C. U., Hillis, A. E., Josephs, K. A., Boeve, B. F., Kertesz, A., Seeley, W. W., Rankin, K. P., Johnson, J. K., Gorno-Tempini, M.-L., Rosen, H., ... Miller, B. L. (2011). Sensitivity of revised diagnostic criteria for the behavioural variant of frontotemporal dementia. *Brain, 134*(9), 2456-2477. https://doi.org/10.1093/brain/awr179

Riedijk, S. R., De Vugt, M. E., Duivenvoorden, H. J., Niermeijer, M. F., Van Swieten, J. C., Verhey, F. R., & Tibben, A. (2006). Caregiver burden, health-related quality of life and coping in dementia caregivers: A comparison of frontotemporal dementia and Alzheimer's disease. *Dementia and Geriatric Cognitive Disorders, 22*(5-6), 405-412. https://doi.org/10.1159/000095750

Schulz, R., & Beach, S. R. (1999). Caregiving as a risk factor for mortality: The Caregiver Health Effects Study. *JAMA, 282*(23), 2215-2219. https://doi.org/10.1001/jama.282.23.2215

Social Security Administration. (2023). *Compassionate Allowances: Conditions.* https://www.ssa.gov/compassionateallowances/conditions.htm

Sollberger, M., Stanley, C. M., Wilson, S. M., Gyurak, A., Beckman, V., Growdon, M., Jang, J., Weiner, M. W., Miller, B. L., & Rankin, K. P. (2009). Neural basis of interpersonal traits in neurodegenerative diseases. *Neuropsychologia, 47*(13), 2812-2827. https://doi.org/10.1016/j.neuropsychologia.2009.06.006

Svanberg, E., Stott, J., & Spector, A. (2010). "Just helping": Children living with a parent with young onset dementia.

Aging and Mental Health, 14(6), 740-751. https://doi.org/10.1080/13607861003713174

Talerico, K. A., & Evans, L. K. (2001). Responding to safety issues in frontotemporal dementias. *Neurology, 56*(Suppl 4), S52-S55. https://doi.org/10.1212/WNL.56.suppl_4.S52

Tsai, R. M., & Boxer, A. L. (2014). Treatment of frontotemporal dementia. *Current Treatment Options in Neurology, 16*(11), 319. https://doi.org/10.1007/s11940-014-0319-0

Volkmer, A., Walton, H., Swinburn, K., Spector, A., Warren, J. D., & Beeke, S. (2023). Results from a randomised controlled pilot study of the Better Conversations with Primary Progressive Aphasia (BCPPA) communication partner training program for people with PPA and their communication partners. *Pilot and Feasibility Studies, 9*(1), 87. https://doi.org/10.1186/s40814-023-01301-6

Made in the USA
Monee, IL
04 November 2026

67383139R00118